WHAT TO DO:

1. Give the following instructions:
   - Apply 10-15 minutes before sexual intercourse deep into the vagina, at the cervical opening while lying down. Use an applicator if using jelly or cream. Effectiveness lasts for one to two hours.
   - The woman should not get up and walk around once the spermicide is in place.
   - Follow the manufacturers' instructions as these can vary according to the preparation being used.

DO NOT DOUCHE AFTER SEXUAL INTERCOURSE AS THIS WILL WASH AWAY THE SPERMICIDE.

Diaphragm and cervical cap

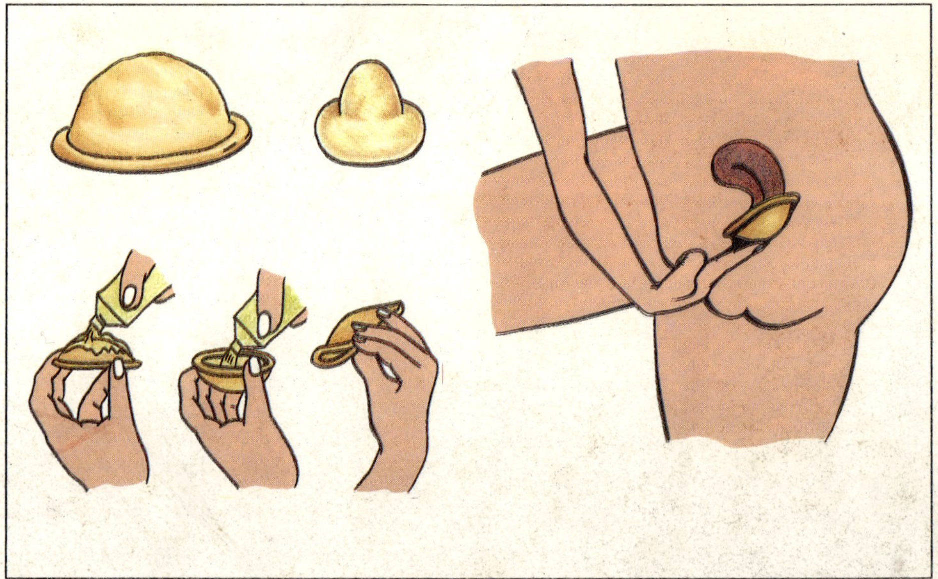

Figure 9. Diaphragm and cervical cap

ACTION:

Prevents pregnancy by blocking the entrance of the sperm to the uterus. The spermicide that is used with it also inactivates or kills sperms.

DESCRIPTION	ADVANTAGES	DISADVANTAGES
• circular, dome shaped rubber disc with a firm rim • inserted into the vagina to cover the cervix and block the entrance of sperm • available in different sizes and styles • used with spermicide	• can be used as a backup method • appropriate for women who have sexual intercourse infrequently	• high failure rate • not appropriate for first sexual intercourse, or women who are prone to urinary tract infection

CONTRAINDICATIONS:

Chronic cervicitis and presence of genital abnormalities which may interfere with insertion.

WHAT TO DO:

1. Ensure proper fit before dispensing a diaphragm or a cap. If it cannot be fitted because of abnormalities in the genital tract, suggest that another method is used.
2. Teach the client the proper way to insert and remove the diaphragm or cap.
3. Give the following instructions:
   - Wash hands carefully with soap and water before handling the diaphragm or cervical cap.
   - Always use with a spermicide. Apply it to both sides of the diaphragm or cap before insertion.
   - Make sure that it is in place before sexual intercourse.
   - Leave it in place until six hours after sexual intercourse. If sexual intercourse is to take place more than once during the six-hour period, leave the diaphragm or cap in place and apply more spermicide with an applicator before each act of intercourse.
   - Do not leave a diaphragm inside the vagina for more than 24 hours, or a cervical cap for more than 36 hours.
   - Do not use it during menstruation or when there is any abnormal vaginal discharge.
   - Do not use it for the first 12 weeks postpartum.
   - To avoid deterioration, take care of the diaphragm or cap by:
     (a) washing it with soap and water after use and drying it with a clean towel before putting it in its case;
     (b) storing it in a cool, dry place;
     (c) checking it for tears or holes every time it is used; and
     (d) using only a water-soluble lubricant with it such as K-Y jelly (petroleum-based lubricants can damage rubber).

☞ ***WOMEN WHO USE A DIAPHRAGM OR CAP SHOULD NOT DOUCHE FOR AT LEAST SIX HOURS AFTER INTERCOURSE.***

Spermicide

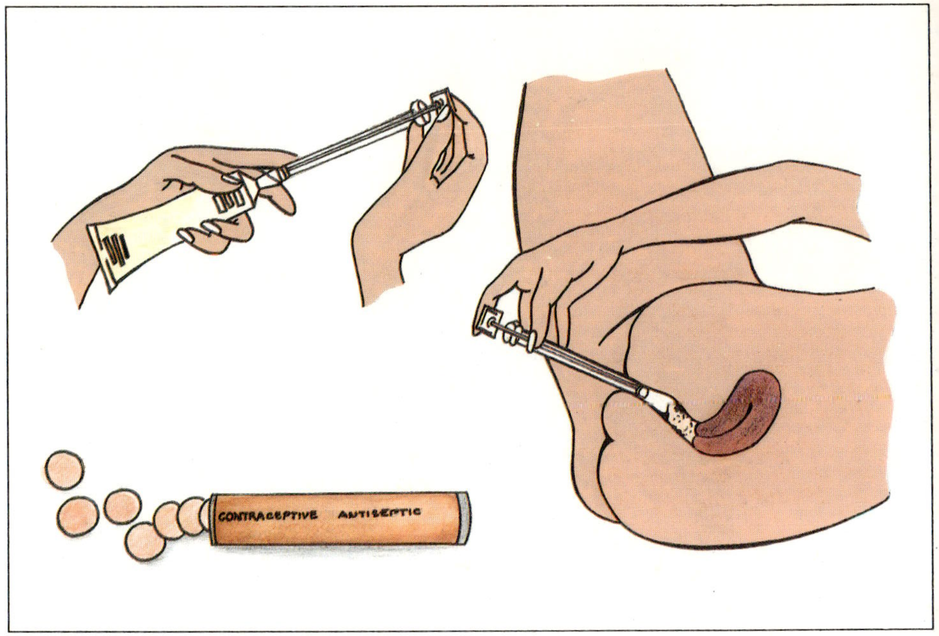

Figure 10. Applying the Spermicide into the vagina with an applicator

ACTION:

Prevents pregnancy by inactivating or killing the sperms.

DESCRIPTION	ADVANTAGES	DISADVANTAGES
• chemical that is applied into the vagina • available in foams, suppositories, tablets, jellies and creams • for better protection, it is also used with a diaphragm, a cervical cap or a condom	• provides some degree of protection against sexually transmitted infections. • can be used as a backup method	• high failure rate • may cause genital irritation and or allergic reactions

QUALITY HEALTH CARE for the ELDERLY

A MANUAL FOR INSTRUCTORS OF NURSES AND OTHER HEALTH WORKERS

Course for Health Care of the Elderly
World Health Organization
Regional Office for the Western Pacific
Manila, Philippines

The World Health Organization is a specialized agency of the United Nations with primary responsibility for international health matters and public health. Through this organization, which was created in 1948, the health professions of 189 countries exchange their knowledge and experience with the aim of making possible the attainment by all citizens of the world by the year 2000 of a level of health that will permit them to lead a socially and economically productive life.

By means of direct technical cooperation with its Member States, and by stimulating such cooperation among them, WHO promotes the development of comprehensive health services, the prevention and control of diseases, the improvement of environmental conditions, the development of human resources for health, the coordination and development of biomedical and health services research, and the planning and implementation of health programmes.

These broad fields of endeavour encompass a wide variety of activities, such as developing systems of primary health care that reach the whole population of Member countries; promoting the health of mothers and children; combating malnutrition; controlling malaria and other communicable diseases including tuberculosis and leprosy; coordinating the global strategy for the prevention and control of AIDS; having achieved the eradication of smallpox, promoting mass immunization against a number of other preventable diseases; improving mental health: providing safe water supplies; and training health personnel of all categories.

Progress towards better health throughout the world also demands international cooperation in such matters as establishing standards for biological substances, pesticides and pharmaceuticals; formulating environmental health criteria; recommending international nonproprietary names for drugs; administering the International Health Regulations; revising the International Statistical Classification of Diseases and Related Health Problems; and collecting and disseminating health statistical information.

Reflecting the concerns and priorities of the Organization and its Member States, WHO publications provide authoritative information and guidance aimed at promoting and protecting health and preventing and controlling disease.

WHO Library Cataloguing in Publication Data

Quality health care for the elderly: a manual for instructors for nurses and other health workers

(Western Pacific Education in Action Series ; no. 6)

1. Health services for the aged - handbooks. 2. Education, Nursing 3. Health personnel - education.

ISBN 92 9061 136 7

CONTENTS

Foreword
Introduction

FOREWORD

The number of people aged 60 years and over in this Region will rapidly increase during the next few decades. It is expected that almost one-third of the people in the world aged 60 years and over will reside in this Region by 2025. Consequently, the need for health services for the elderly will be a growing regional issue.

The primary concern of the World Health Organization is for the improvement of the well-being and quality of life of the elderly, not merely the extension of their life expectancy. To achieve this goal, adequate preventive, curative and rehabilitative services must be provided to the elderly.

Until recently, many countries in the Region have paid little specific attention to the health care of the elderly. The primary responsibility to care for the elderly has been left to family members. In those countries, few health workers are equipped with sufficient specialized knowledge on health care of the elderly. The increased need for health services for the elderly and the weakening of traditional family ties emphasize the important role of health workers as formal service providers for the elderly. If health workers are not equipped with appropriate skills and knowledge, it will not be possible to provide adequate health services to the elderly.

The main objective of this manual is therefore to provide instructors of health workers with up-to-date information on these skills and the knowledge necessary for good health care of elderly people. This manual is not intended to cover all aspects of the health care of the elderly, rather, it suggests a framework for instruction. Therefore, instructors of health schools/institutions in various countries are encouraged to modify or add other useful information according to their national situations and cultural beliefs and values.

I hope this manual will stimulate and facilitate the development of well-trained health personnel in the field of health of the elderly, resulting in improved quality of life for all.

S.T. Han, MD, Ph.D.
Regional Director

INTRODUCTION

More people are reaching old age than ever before. Therefore, all primary health care workers are beginning to encounter many older persons in their daily work. And because most of the health workers who provide services to older persons are not at that stage of life themselves and therefore have no firsthand knowledge of the experience (Saxon & Etten, 1987), it is necessary to gain an understanding through educational methods of reading, lecture, practical exercises, and clinical field work.

The overall *goal* of this course is to educate health care workers in strategies which *promote health and wellness of the elderly.*

This manual has been written for instructors who are responsible for the training of nurses and other primary health care workers. It is suitable for preservice as well as postgraduate curricula.

Please note five important ideas in regard to this manual:

1. The information on aging contained in this course *is meant to be incorporated into the daily clinical practice of many types of health care facilities.*

2. It is *not* intended as a training manual to develop geriatrics as a seperate subspecialty.

3. The bibliographies are extensive and are *not* required reading. The course content is based on these references and stands on its own.

4. Only selected (that is the most common) problems of aging are included as alterations to the normal age-related changes. *Instructors are kindly asked to refer to other sources for illnesses and diseases which they choose to emphasize beyond the ones included, since these can be found in any good general medical-surgical text.*

5. Some modules are considerably shorter than others. Instructors may wish to present two shorter ones together on a single day.

The contents of the course are modelled on, and some entire sections actually taken directly from, the WHO document titled "Strengthening the Teaching of Diarrhoeal Diseases in Basic Training Programmes: A Manual for Instructors of Nurses and Other Health Workers" (WHO Field Test 1992, Programme for the Control of Diarrhoeal Disease (CDD), WHO, 1211 Geneva 27 Switzerland). The Quality Health Care for the Elderly curriculum (see pages 4-8 of the section on Curriculum) outlines the course of study. Using materials from other sections in the manual, instructors can develop lesson plans on the topics listed on the curriculum plans. The manual also contains evaluation strategies to assess competency.

Acknowledgement

This activity is initiated by the World Health Organization, Western Pacific Regional Office with funding from the Transfer of Technology Project sponsored by the Government of Japan.

Christine Sheehy is acknowledged for preparation of the manuscript which lead to this document. She is a Professor of Nursing and Program Director of the Master's level Geriatric Nurse Practitioner course at the College of Nursing, University of Arizona, Tucson, USA. While gerontologists often focus on care and illness, Professor Sheehy is distinguished for emphasizing the importance of human vitality and the control of life of the elderly.

COVER PHOTO BY KOH KOK HWA

Curriculum

CURRICULUM

Curriculum objectives

The curriculum plans in this section outline the course of study designed to help students learn about health care interventions for older persons. Students who complete this course should be able to:

- explain the reasons for needing to learn more about the special needs of older persons;
- define quality health care for the elderly;
- understand the concept of "stereotypes" and the importance of overcoming them;
- describe some of the current theories which have been proposed to explain the process of aging;
- describe normal age-related changes and the implications of these;
- screen for normal age-related decrements and assess, identify and prioritize alterations, and develop care plans with goals and interventions, and ways of evaluating their effectiveness;
- identify common health problems (that is deviations from expected age-related changes), develop plans of care with goals and interventions, and ways of evaluating the effectiveness;
- describe changes in the reproductive systems of men and women, relate changes to needs for sexuality among older adults, and apply knowledge about sexuality in later years by developing plans with goals and interventions and ways of evaluating effectiveness;
- describe current explanations for the cause and progression of Alzheimer's disease and apply knowledge by developing plans with goals and interventions and ways of evaluating effectiveness;
- describe influences of cultural background on the provision of mental health support to older adults and their families, identify the most common mental health problems, summarize information about group strategies most frequently used to maintain and/or restore the emotional well-being of older persons and apply knowledge by developing plans with goals and interventions and ways of evaluating effectiveness;
- explain the concept of "caregiver burden", describe risks to older persons and families that result from sustained and unrelieved caregiver burden,

recognize mistreatment of the elderly, and develop plans of care with goals and interventions for caregiver support and ways of evaluating the effectiveness;

- describe needs for health promotion in older persons, including sleep and exercise, nutrition, screening, case-finding and referral, prevention of smoking and alcohol abuse, accident prevention and medication management;
- enumerate strategies for health promotion in regard to health promotion needs; and
- develop a health promotion programme for a community and ways of evaluating programme effectiveness.

Components of the curriculum plan

The curriculum plan is organized according to topics and divided into (1) time, (2) learning objectives, (3) teaching/learning materials, and (4) student assessment.

(1) ***Time*** required to cover each topic. The instructor may need to increase or decrease the suggested time. For example, when the class is large, more time will be needed for the exercises.

(2) ***Learning objectives*** for each topic. These state in behavioural terms what the student is expected to know and be able to do after completing each module, and, after completing the course of study about quality health care for the elderly. The learning domains may be **cognitive** (that is knowledge), **affective** (that is concerning change of attitude) and in some cases as with assessment skills, both cognitive and **psychomotor** (that is learning which involves hands-on clinical experience).

(3) ***Teaching and learning materials*** for the instructor and students to use.

- The *entire* contents of this manual are for the instructor.
- *Course modules* which contain the basic information to be learned should be given to students.
- Approaches and materials are recommended to enhance the learning experience. However, instructors are encouraged to use the basic exercises and strategies as a guide, to build upon them based on their own experience, and to individualize learning experiences as appropriate to the culture and setting.

- Lively, "*getting to know you*" group interaction exercises are encouraged prior to the teaching activity(ies).

(4) ***Student assessent activities*** can be used to measure student progress in achieving the learning objectives. Assessment may be *formal* such as by the multiple choice examinations proposed (see Examination questions on page 23-45 of the Student assessment tools section). The instructor may also use an assessment checklist to observe students conducting an assessment during a field visit (see Assessment of practical skills on pages 1-22 of the Student evaluation tools section). However, the instructor can also assess progress more *informally* by reading the student's answers to individual exercises in a course module or by observing the student during a role-play exercise.

NOTE: ***It is NOT necessary for every one of these assessment activities to be used for every module. Questions to determine knowledge gained appear as exercises at the end of each module as well as in the examination section as multiple choice questions. They are included for instructor convenience. If, for example, an instructor prefers not to use the multiple choice test, the instructor should feel free to add additional short-answer exercises or whatever is felt to be better suited to his or her teaching style.***

Quality Health Care for the Elderly (QHCE) Curriculum

Module	Time	Learning objectives	Teaching/learning	Student assessment
1. Overview	3 to 5 hours	1. Explain the reasons for needing to learn more about the special needs of older persons; 2. Define quality health care for the elderly; 3. Understand the concept of "stereotypes" and the importance of overcoming them; and 4. Describe some of the current theories which have been proposed to explain the process of aging.	Audiovisual aids to illustrate content as desired. Didactic, group discussion techniques.	Response to Exercise A. Answers to short-answer exercises 1 and 2. Answers to Module 1 examination questions.
2. The senses	5 to 10 hours	1. Describe the normal age-related changes which occur in the senses and the implication of these: • skin • vision • hearing • taste • smell • touch, sensation, and balance 2. Screen for normal age-related sensory decrements: • assess all senses • identify and prioritize alteration • develop care plans including goals and interventions for education and safety 3. Identify common health problems, (that is deviations from expected age-related changes in the senses); and 4. Develop care plan (with goals and interventions) for common problems and ways of evaluating the effectiveness.	Ex. : Guidelines) all Ex. : Care Plans) in the List: Nursing Diagnosis) module Substances for assessment skills; **taste**, e.g. lemon juice, salt, sugar, mint; **smell**, e.g. peanut butter, cloves, oranges, coffee, tea; **sight**, hand-held Snellen Chart (in jacket) at the end of this manual to be provided to students; and Didactic, group discussion, demonstration, and/or return demonstration.	Responses to Exercises A and B. Answers to short-answer exercises 1 and 2. Answers to Module 2 examination questions. Assessment of practical skills

Quality Health Care for the Elderly (QHCE) Curriculum (Cont'd)

Module	Time	Learning objectives	Teaching/learning	Student assessment
3. The musculo-skeletal system	3 to 5 hours	1. Describe normal age-related changes which occur in muscles, bones and supporting structures; 2. Recognize the most common musculoskeletal problems and diseases of older persons; 3. Detail strategies for safety and health promotion in regard to changes in the musculoskeletal system; and 4. Identify symptoms of osteoarthritis, and develop a plan of care (with goals and interventions) and ways of evaluating the effectiveness of the plan.	A/V aids or models as appropriate. Didactic group discussion, demonstration, return demonstration, role-play.	Responses to Exercises A and B. Answers to short-answer exercises 1, 2 and 3. Answers to Module 3 examination questions. Assessment of practical skills.
4. The urinary system	5 to 7 hours	1. Describe normal age-related changes which occur in the urinary system; 2. Screen the urinary system for normal age-related function: • assess system • identify and prioritize alterations • develop care plans including goals and interventions for health promotion strategies; 3. Identify common health problems, (that is deviations from expected age-related changes) in the urinary system; and 4. Develop plans (with goals and interventions) for common problems, and ways of evaluating effectiveness.	A/V aids or models as appropriate. Didactic, group discussion, demonstration, return demonstration, role-play.	Responses to Exercises A and B. Answers to short-answer exercises 1 and 2. Answers to Module 4 examination questions. Assessment of practical skills.

Quality Health Care for the Elderly (QHCE) Curriculum (Cont'd)

Module	Time	Learning objectives	Teaching/learning	Student assessment
5. The gastro-intestinal system	2 to 4 hours	1. Describe normal age-related changes which occur in the gastrointestinal (GI) system; 2. Screen the GI system for normal age-related function: • assess system • identify and assign priority to any dysfunction • develop care plans including goals and interventions for health promotion strategies; 3. Identify common health problems, (that is deviations from expected age-related changes) in the gastrointestinal system; and 4. Develop plans (with goals and interventions) for common problems, and ways of evaluating effectiveness.	A/V aids or models as appropriate. Didactic group discussion, demonstration, return demonstration, role-play.	Response to Exercises A and B. Answers to short-answer exercises 1 and 2. Answers to Module 5 examination questions. Assessment of practical skills.
6. The Cardio-vascular and respira-tory systems	2 to 4 hours	1. Describe normal age-related changes which occur in the cardiovascular and respiratory systems; 2. List common health problems, (that is deviations from expected age-related changes) in the cardiovascular and respiratory systems; and 3. Develop plans (with goals and interventions) for the management of such common health problems; and 4. Develop plans (with goals and interventions) for health promotion for cardiopulmonary fitness.	A/V aids and anatomical models to illustrate content as desired. Didactic, group discussions, role-play demonstration, and/or return demonstration.	Response to Exercise A. Answers to short-answer exercises 1 and 2. Answers to Module 6 examination questions. Assessment of practical skills.
7. Age-related changes in the reproduc-tive system and late life sexuality	5 to 7 hours	1. Describe normal age-related changes which occur in the reproductive systems of men and women; 2. Relate these changes to needs for sexuality among older adults; and 3. Apply knowledge about sexuality in later years by developing a plan (with goals and interventions for teaching), and ways of evaluating effectiveness.	A/V aids and anatomical models to illustrate context as desired. Didactive, group discussions, role-play, demonstrations, and/or return demonstrations.	Response to Exercise A and B. Answers to short-answer exercises 1 and 2. Answers to Module 7 examination questions.

Quality Health Care for the Elderly (QHCE) Curriculum (Cont'd)

Module	Time	Learning objectives	Teaching/learning	Student assessment
8. Endocrine and immune function	2 to 4 hours	1. Describe (selected) normal age-related changes which occur in the endocrine and immune function; and 2. Apply knowledge about non-insulin dependent diabetes mellitus (NIDDM) by developing a plan (with goals and interventions for teaching) for the disease, and ways of evaluating effectiveness.	A/V aids or anatomical models as appropriate. Didactic, group discussion, role-play, demonstration and return demonstration.	Response to Exercise A. Answers to (one) short-answer exercise. Answers to Module 8 examination questions. Assessment of practical skills.
9. Dementing illness and changes in the brain	2 to 5 hours	1. Explain age-related changes which occur in the brain; 2. Describe current explanations for the cause and progression of Alzheimer's disease; and 3. Develope a plan (with goals and interventions) for older persons with this problem, and ways of evaluating effectiveness.	Didactic, group discussion, role-play	Response to Exercises A and B. Answers to (one) short-answer exercise. Answers to Module 9 examination questions. Assessment of practical skills.
10. Mental health and aging	4 to 6 hours	1. Describe (selected) influences of cultural background on the provision of mental health support to older adults and their families; 2. Identify the most common mental health problems of older adults; 3. Apply knowledge about depression by developing a care plan (with goals and interventions) and ways for evaluating the effectiveness; and 4. Summarize information about group strategies which are most frequently used to maintain and/or restore emotional well-being of older persons.	Didactic group discussion, interview (simulated), role-play.	Response to Exercises A and B. Answers to short-answer exercises 1 and 2. Answers to Module 10 examination questions.

Quality Health Care for the Elderly (QHCE) Curriculum (Cont'd)

Module	Time	Learning objectives	Teaching/learning	Student assessment
11. Supporting families in caregiving	4 to 6 hours	1. Explain the concept of "caregiver burden"; 2. Describe risks to older persons and families that result from sustained and unrelieved caregiver burden; 3. Recognize mistreatment of the elderly; and 4. Develop care plans (with goals and interventions) for caregiver support and ways of evaluating the effectiveness.	Didactic group discussion, role-play.	Response to Exercises A and B. Answers to short-answer exercises 1 and 2. Answers to Module 11 examination questions.
12. Health promotion summary	4 to 6 hours	1. Describe needs for health promotion in older persons including sleep and exercise, nutrition, screening, case-finding and referral, prevention of smoking and alcohol abuse, accident prevention and medication management; 2. Enumerate health promotion in regard to the needs; and 3. Develop a health promotion programme for a community, and ways of evaluating programme effectiveness.	Didactic, group discussion, role-play	Response to Exercise B. Answers to short-answer exercises 1, 2, and 3. Answers to Module 12 examination questions. Assessment of practical skills.

Methods

METHODS

This section of the manual describes a variety of teaching methods for helping students learn the topics on the Quality Health Care for the Elderly Curriculum (pages 4-8 of the Curriculum section). This section also suggests ways to solve problems the instructor may find while trying to use the suggested teaching methods.

- Providing course modules
- Selecting appropriate teaching methods
- Guidelines for using active teaching methods

Providing course modules

Twelve course modules are included in this manual: (1) Overview; (2) The senses; (3) The musculoskeletal system; (4) The urinary system; (5) The gastrointestinal system; (6) The cardiovascular and respiratory systems; (7) Age-related changes in the reproductive system and late life sexuality; (8) Endocrine and immune function; (9) Dementing illness and changes in the brain; (10) Mental health and aging; (11) Supporting families in caregiving; and (12) Health promotion summary.

The course modules provide student readings, individual written exercises, group discussion topics, case studies, and other activities. Using these instructional methods is easier when each student has their own copy of the modules. For this reason it is worthwhile trying to get enough copies.

Selecting appropriate teaching methods

People learn in three basic ways by:

- receiving **information**,
- seeing an **example**, and
- **practising**.

The table on the following page shows some common teaching methods for providing information, examples, and practice to help students learn. These methods are used in the course modules in this manual.

	To provide	Use such methods as:	Learner participates by:
Less Active	Information	1. Lecture 2. Student reading	Hearing
	Examples	3. Demonstration 4. Pictures and slides 5. Video cassette	Seeing
More Active	Practice	6. Role-play exercise 7. Small group activity 8. Written exercise 9. Case study 10. Individual feedback 11. Supervised practice in field visits and placements	Doing

Lectures and reading assignments are useful for introducing new information. However, methods that involve students more actively, such as role–plays and supervised practice, are more likely to be effective in helping students understand, remember, and correctly do what they have learned.

Sometimes the schedule, class size, or other factors might not permit use of the teaching method recommended in the module. The instructor will then need to select an alternative.

The table on the following pages lists the advantages and disadvantages of using each of the methods as a guide for choosing an appropriate alternative. For example, a class may be too large for the instructor to evaluate written exercises and also give frequent individual feedback. Therefore, the instructor will need to select another active method to provide practice and feedback. For example, if role-plays are appropriate to use to practice a skill, the instructor may be able to observe students in role-plays in small groups and encourage feedback among the students themselves.

Teaching methods and educational media		
To provide	**Advantages**	**Disadvantages**
Information	**1. Lecture** • Saves time (for the teacher) and resources when introducing new content. • Reaches a large group of students.	• Promotes passive learning. • Does not facilitate problem-solving. • Offers almost no chance to check learning progress. • Offers no chance for individual learning pace. • Does not permit practice of skills.
	2. Student reading • Allows the student to work at his or her own pace. • Can be assigned as homework, freeing classroom time for discussion, demonstration and practical work.	• Does not encourage students to share ideas. • May be costly if modules are not provided and have to be reproduced.
Examples	**3. Demonstration** • Ensures closer contact with concrete problems. • Facilitates acquisition of practical, intellectual communication skills. • Enables logical step-by-step presentation of correct way of doing a task. • Allows questions from students. • Reduces damage to equipment and material when students do practical work afterwards.	• Serves only a limited number of students at a time. • Promotes relatively passive learning (except for when students can repeat the demonstration). • Offers little possibility to check learning process. • Offers no chance for individual learning pace. • Does not permit practice of skills.
	4. Pictures and slides • Are suitable for large audiences (slides) or small groups (pictures). • Are relatively easy to produce and (in black and white) reproduce. • Are the least expensive of the current forms of visual media. • Are easily adaptable to self-learning packages. • Pictures do not need special equipment.	• Do not permit sharing of good ideas and problems. • Test knowledge, not practical skills. • Require good light for viewing pictures. • May not be suitable to large groups (especially true of photographs). • Requires electricity.
	5. Video cassette • Offers sight, sound, and movement of real situation, when patients are not available. • Is suitable for large audiences. • Conveys more information in less time than real situation by compressing time and space. • Can help develop attitudes, pose problems, demonstrate skills, and provide some skill practice in making decisions.	• Does not permit self-pacing. • Is difficult and costly to produce and reproduce. • Requires electricity. • Depends on equipment that may not be available and may be difficult to transport

Teaching methods and educational media (cont'd)		
To provide	**Advantages**	**Disadvantages**
Practice	**6. Role-play exercise** • Provides an opportunity, in a controlled situation, to develop communications and other practical skills. • Gives students a chance to develop empathy and understanding by being in "someone else's shoes". • Facilitates evaluation and feedback.	• Is time-consuming. • Depends on student's imagination and willingness to participate.
	7. Small group activity • Permits instructor-student and student-student dialogue. • Facilitates evaluation and feedback.	• Is a costly use of personnel and time (unless peer teaching is used).
	8. Written exercise (short answer exercise, sample examination questions, etc.) • Reinforces and tests understanding of theoretical knowledge. • Allows self-pacing. • Obliges students to work things out for themsellves. • Permits self-evaluation. • Facilitates evaluation and feedback. • Is easy to use.	• Does not encourage students to share ideas, problems and questions. • Tests knowledge, but not practical skills.
	9. Case study • Gives students opportunity to apply their knowledge. • Helps develop decision-making skills. • May be used to identify problems. • Facilitates evaluation and feedback.	• Promotes acquisition of knowledge and decision-making skills, but not practical, behavioural skills.
	10. Individual feedback • Is tailored to individual needs. • Ensures that everyone understands. • Permits problems to be immediately identified and solved.	• Is a costly use of personnel and time (unless peer feedback is given). • Can be done only when other students are occupied with work.
	11. Supervised practice field visits and field placements • Provides an active learning and practice situation. • Permits evaluation of degree to which educational objectives (practical skills) have been attained. • Develops qualities of observation and decision-making. • Ensures closer contact with reality (professional, health situation of a community, colleagues and teachers)	• Is a costly use of personnel, transportation and materials. • Covers only a limited group of students at one time and place. • Sometimes puts the patient in a difficult situation. • Is difficult to standardize quality of learning experience. • Requires careful planning. • Depends on quality of supervision available in the field.

Teaching methods and educational media (cont'd)		
To provide	**Advantages**	**Disadvantages**
Practice	**11. Supervised practice field visits and field placements (cont'd)** • Permits comparison between practice and theory. • Promotes development of self-confidence. • Facilitates evaluation and feedback	

Adapted from Educational Handbook for Health Personnel, 6th Edition, By JJ. Gilbert, WHO Offset Publication No. 35; World Health Organization, Geneva, Switzerland, 342-345, 1987.

Guidelines for using active teaching methods

This section provides the instructor with guidelines on how to use some of the recommended active teaching methods.

General techniques for motivating students

Encourage interaction

During the first day or two, interact at least once with every student and encourage each one to interact with you frequently. This will help students to overcome possible shyness and encourage them to participate actively throughout the course.

Look carefully, as frequently as possible, at each student's work (including answers to short-answer exercises). Check to see if students are having any problems, even if they do not ask for help. If you show interest and give each student some undivided attention, he or she will feel more compelled to do the work. Also, if the students know that the instructor is interested in what they are doing, they are more likely to ask for help when they need it.

Be readily available to students at all times: remain in the room and look approachable. Do not do other work.

***Keep participants* involved**

Frequently ask questions of students to check their understanding and to keep them actively thinking and participating. Questions that begin with "what", "why", or "how" require more than just a few words to answer. Avoid questions that can be answered with just one word (for example, questions that begin with "Do you...?")

One way to encourage participants

The following approach can prompt everyone's participation in answering a question. It is particularly appropriate when the expected answer is a short list of items, such as a group of activities.

1) Ask the question. Tell students to think about two or more answers and write them down.
2) When most students are ready, have students call out their answers.
3) Record the answers on a flip chart or chalkboard. At this time, do not evaluate the answers. Simply record them.
4) When all students have contributed, review the list with the group, crossing out repeat items and combining items which students agree are similar. The discussion should be limited to clarifying what particular items mean and their benefits.

After asking a question, *pause*. Give students time to think of an answer. A common mistake is when the instructor asks a question and then answers it himself or herself. If no one answers your question, rephrasing it can help to break the tension of silence. But do not do this repeatedly; some silence is productive.

Acknowledge all student responses. This will help students feel valued and will encourage them to continue to participate. Do this with a comment, a "thank you" or a definite nod. If you think the student has missed the point, ask for clarification or ask if another student has a suggestion. If a student feels his or her comments are ridiculed or ignored, they may withdraw from the discussion entirely or not speak voluntarily again.

Answer students' questions willingly, and encourage them to ask questions when they have them rather than to hold the questions until a later time.

Address students by name when you call on them, and when you give them credit or thanks. Use the speaker's name when you refer back to a previous comment.

Always maintain eye contact with students so everyone feels included. Be careful not to always look at the same students. Looking at a student for even a few seconds will often prompt a reply, even from a shy and quiet person.

Keep the session lively and focused

Keep your presentation lively by:

- presenting information conversationally instead of reading it.
- moving around the room and using natural hand gestures;

- speaking clearly and varying the pace and pitch of your voice; and
- using a variety of methods to present information, such as written materials, writing on a board or flip-chart, demonstration, lecture and discussion.

Write key ideas on a flip-chart or chalk board as they are offered. This is a good way to acknowledge responses. The speaker will know his or her suggestion has been heard and will have the satisfaction of seeing it recorded for the entire group.

When recording ideas on a flip-chart, use the student's own words, if possible. If the student's response is too long, reword the idea and check it with the student before writing it. You want to be sure the student feels you understand and are recording the idea accurately.

Do not turn your back to the group for long periods as you write.

Paraphrase and summarize frequently to keep students focused on a clear idea and to keep discussions on track. Ask students to clarify their statements, if necessary. Also, encourage other students to ask a speaker to repeat or clarify the speaker's statement.

Restate the original question to the group to focus attention on the main issue. If you feel someone will resist getting back on track, first pause to get the group's attention. Tell them they have strayed from the point then restate the original question.

Do not let several students talk at the same time. When this happens, stop the talkers and assign an order for speaking. (For example, say, "Let's hear John's comment first, then Salvador's, then Maria's.") People usually will not interrupt if they know they will have a turn to talk.

Thank students whose comments are brief and to the point.

Try to encourage the quieter students to talk. Ask to hear from a student who has not spoken before, or walk towards someone to focus attention on them and make them feel that they are being asked to talk.

Manage discussion problems

Manage the student who talks too much, for example, by:

- walking towards the student when they are talking to make them feel self-conscious. Then walk away from the student or turn your back to to focus attention away from the student and move the discussion on to another speaker;
- breaking in quickly when the student pauses and ask to hear from another member of the group;

- recording the student's main idea on a flip-chart. As they continue to talk about the idea, point to it on the flip-chart or chalk board and say, "Thank you, we have already covered your suggestion." Then ask the group for another idea; and

- not asking the talkative student any more questions. If they answer all the questions directed to the group, ask for an answer from another individual specifically or from a specific subgroup. (For example, ask, "Does anyone on this side of the table have an idea?")

Try to identify students who have difficulty understanding or speaking the language. Speak slowly and distinctly so you can be more easily understood, and encourage these students to communicate. If necessary, speak with the student in their native language to clarify a point.

Reinforce student efforts

As an instructor, you will have your own style of interacting with students. However, you can positively reinforce students' efforts by:

- avoiding the use of facial expressions or comments that could cause students to feel ridiculed;

- sitting or bending down to be on the same level as a student when talking individually to them;

- not answering hurriedly;

- encouraging students to speak to you by allowing them time; and

- appearing interested, saying, "That's a good question/suggestion".

> Reinforce students who:
>
> ◊ try hard;
>
> ◊ ask for an explanation of a confusing point;
>
> ◊ do a good job on an exercise;
>
> ◊ participate in group discussions; and
>
> ◊ help other students (without distracting them by talking at length about irrelevant matters).

Helping individuals do student readings and written exercises

Look available, interested, and ready to help.

Encourage students to ask you questions whenever they need help.

If important issues or questions arise when you are talking with an individual, make note of them to discuss later with the entire group.

If a question arises which you think you cannot answer adequately, get help as soon as possible from another instructor or from the resource materials provided in this manual.

Providing individual feedback

Before the individual feedback session, remind yourself of the purpose of the feedback and the major points to make during the discussion. Also, check in the module to see if there have been any short-answer exercises since the previous discussion.

Compare the student's answer to a short-answer exercise with the answer provided in the module. Compare the student's answer to the individual feedback exercise with the answer sheet. If the answer provided to an exercise is labeled "Possible Answers", the student's answer does not need to match exactly, but should be reasonable. If there is a definite answer provided, be sure the student's answer is correct.

If the student's answer to any exercise is not correct or is not reasonable, ask the student questions to determine why the error was made. For example, a student may not understand certain terms used in the exercise, or may be unable to do a mathematical calculation, or may not understand a basic concept being taught.

Once you have identified the reason(s) for the incorrect answer to an exercise, help the student to correct the problem. For example, if the student has difficulty understanding the concept itself, you might try relating it to situations in the student's own health area. After the student understands the problematic term or concept, ask them to work the exercise or part of the exercise again, to be sure they understand it.

Summarize, or ask students to summarize, what was done in the exercise and why it was done. Emphasize that it is most important to learn and remember the concept or the process demonstrated by the exercise. Give the student a copy of the answer sheet, if one is provided.

Leading a group discussion

Plan to conduct the group discussion at a time when you are very sure all students will have completed the preceding work. Wait to announce this time until most students are ready, so that others will not hurry.

Before beginning the discussion, refer to the appropriate Instructor Guide (provided with the module) to remind yourself of the purpose of the discussion and the major points to make.

Always begin the group discussion by explaining the purpose of the discussion.

Usually there is no single correct answer that needs to be agreed on in a discussion. Just be sure the conclusions of the group are reasonable and that all students understand how the conclusions were reached.

Try to involve most the group members in the discussion. Record key ideas on a flip-chart as they are offered. Keep your participation to a minimum, but ask questions to keep the discussion active and on track.

Always conclude the exercise by asking a student to summarize what was done in the exercise and why it was done. Emphasize that it is most important to learn and remember the concept or the process demonstrated by the exercise. Give students a copy of the answer sheet, if one is provided.

Coordinating a role-play

Before the role-play begins, review the purpose of the role-play, roles to be assigned, background information to provide, issues to be covered, and major points to make in the group discussion to follow the role-play.

As students come to you for instructions before the exercise begins:

- assign roles. At the beginning, select individuals who are outgoing rather than shy, possibly volunteers. If needed, an instructor may set a model for the group by acting in the first role-play.
- explain to participants how role-playing is done. The persons taking the role are given a "script" or part they are to enact. Have them try to imagine how the real person in the role would feel. This helps to make the person taking the role appear more realistic. Students who are not playing the roles are observers. They should make observations, take notes and, when the role-play is concluded, use their notes and observations to comment.
- provide key role-players with any available props appropriate for the exercise.

- encourage role-play participants to periodically get up and move around during the role-play.
- suggest that role-play participants speak clearly and loudly enough for other group members to hear.
- allow preparation time for students who will have a role in the exercise.

When all students are ready for the role-play to begin, arrange seating or placement of participants. If only two or three people will assume roles, situate them apart from the rest of the group. Push the table and chairs aside as needed. If all students in the group will assume a role, have everyone sit in a circle, with or without a table.

Begin by introducing the players in their roles and stating the purpose or situation.

During the role-play, interrupt only if the participants are having tremendous difficulty.

When the role-play is finished, thank the students. Be sure to give considerate feedback to students. Begin by discussing things well done in the role-play, and then discuss ways it could have been improved.

Try to involve all group members in the discussion after the role-play.

Always conclude the exercise by asking students to summarize what they have learned from the role-play.

Relating modules to future jobs

Discuss the application of new concepts to real problems in health facilities. This is the one instructor function that is most likely to ensure that students begin to think about how to apply what they are learning.

Discuss any difficulties students might encounter while trying to implement the skills being learned.

Reinforce students who discuss or ask questions about practical application of skills by acknowledging and responding to their concerns.

Do not reject alternative methods suggested by participants; discuss alternative methods thoughtfully and compare these methods to ones in the module.

Ask questions to encourage students to think about how to apply the concept or process in a health facility.

Reinforce students for their good work, for example, by:

- praising them for the list they compiled; commenting on their understanding of the exercise;
- commenting on their creative or useful suggestions for applying the concept on the job; or
- praising them for their ability to work together as a group.

Bibliography

Teaching of Diarrhoeal Diseases in Basic Training Programme: A Manual for Instructors of Nurses and Other Health Workers. WHO Field Test 1992, Programme for the Control of Diarrhoeal Disease (CDD), WHO, 1211 Geneva 27 Switzerland.

Overview

MODULE 1 - *OVERVIEW*

Objectives

On completion of this module, the student should be able to:

1. explain the reasons for needing to learn more about the special needs of older persons;
2. define quality health care for the elderly;
3. understand the concept of "stereotypes" and the importance of overcoming them; and
4. describe some of the current theories which have been proposed to explain the process of aging.

Why do we need to learn more about the special needs of the elderly?

As a result of advances in medical and health care related sciences, people are living much longer than in the past. In fact, in some countries as much as 10-25% of the population may be over 65 years of age by the years 2010 to 2050. Elimination of the fatal effects of many diseases, such as tuberculosis, rheumatic fever, smallpox, diphtheria, tetanus, polio and pneumonia has contributed to the length of time people live.

The majority of the elderly reside in their local communities and wish to remain there. Health care workers can support them in staying independent and healthy by understanding age-related norms, thereby maximizing the capabilities of older people.

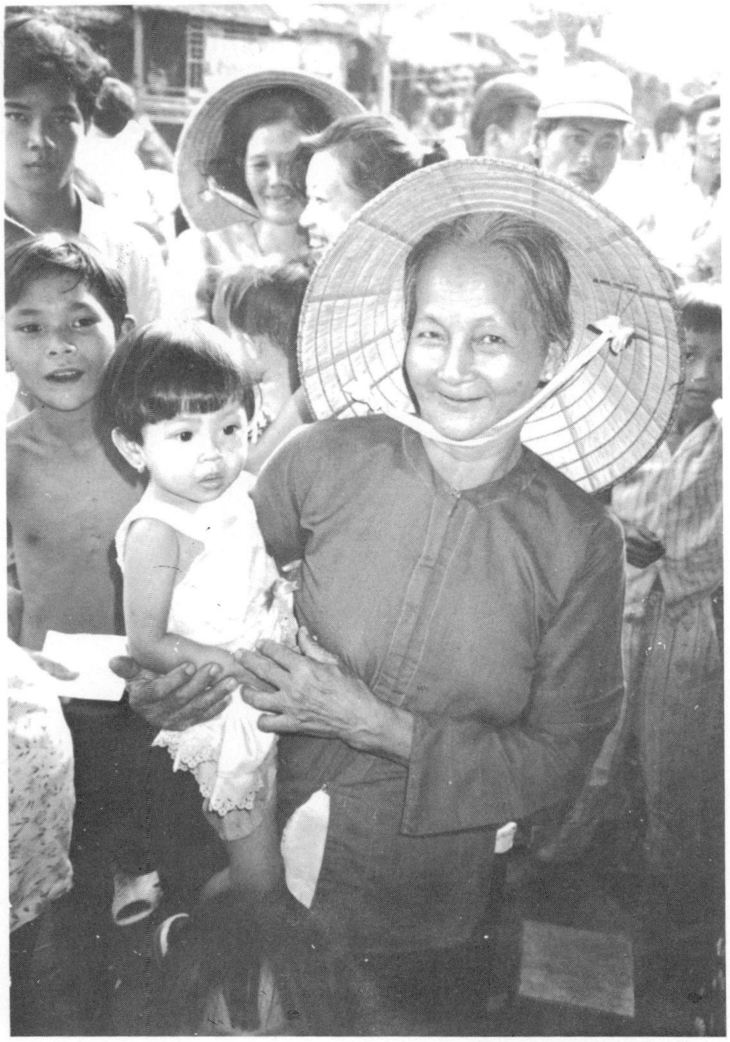

Photo couresy of Dr Bilous

Family responsibilities for the elderly promotes social and mental engagement. In this photo the grandmother ensures that the child is given all routine immunizations.

Early intervention and treatment of chronic illnesses, and instruction in healthy lifestyle habits can also enhance their well-being. Even among those elderly living in the community and considered to be reasonably healthy, there is substantial need for ongoing health care supervision, including coordination and mobilization of resources, monitoring of nutrition, blood pressure and the effectiveness and side effects of routine medications taken.

Knowledge of what is normal in older age, information about ways to promote fitness and awareness of what can be realistically expected as a standard of health, increase the likelihood that older persons can remain vigorous and enjoy a happy old age.

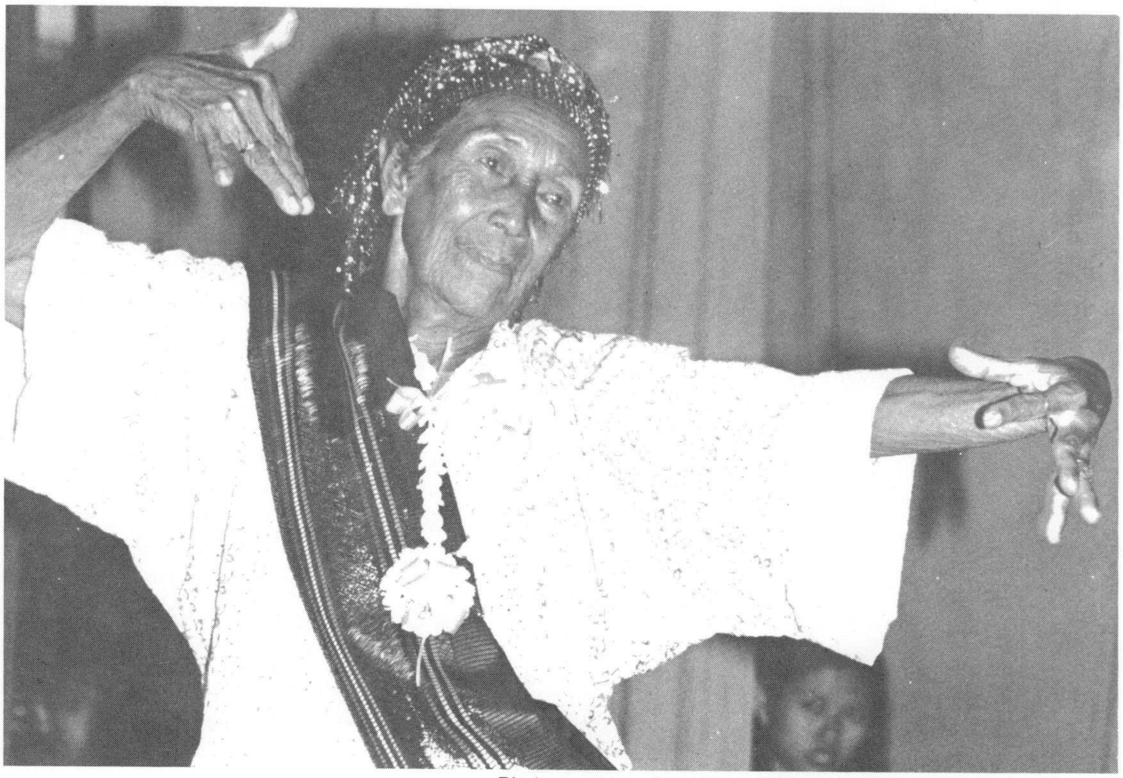

Photo courtesy of Coalition of Services for the Elderly, Inc. (COSE)

Quality care for the elderly promotes maintaining vigour and happiness.

What constitutes quality health care for the elderly?

Quality health care for the elderly is care that is provided by health workers for the purposes of:

- promoting health and minimizing limitations in the elderly,
- maintaining independent lifestyles for the elderly in the familiar surrounding of their communities;
- supporting family members in their efforts to sustain the well-being of their older relatives;
- cooperating to create a community which can provide a comfortable life for the elderly;
- restoring function following an illness when necessary; and
- doing such things with sensitivity to the rights and dignity of older persons.

In order to accomplish these objectives, health workers need to have accurate and current knowledge of the physical processes of aging and related health and social support systems which reinforce preservative and restorative practices.

How do stereotypes apply to the elderly?

Stereotypes are beliefs or generalizations about characteristics or qualities which are felt to be typical of a particular group (Funk & Wagnalls, 1966). For example, you may have heard statements such as "all old people have trouble remembering", or "old people complain all the time", or "old people are all alike", or "all old people are sweet", or "all old people are content". Generally, stereotypical statements result from the absence of factual information or experience with a single event which leads one to incorrect impressions. Stereotyping (having a fixed expectation) about older persons can seriously limit their potential. It is important to overcome these ways of thinking because stereotyping can contribute to discrimination, demoralization, loss of self-esteem, loss of function, inactivity, and physical and mental decline of older persons (Palmore, 1990). Stereotyping also acts to counteract desired, positive interventions for health promotion and quality of life.

What is aging?

Aging refers to the regular changes which occur after the age of physical maturity in persons living under usual environmental conditions, as they advance in years of age. It is not known precisely how or why organisms age but many theories have been proposed to explain the aging process. The major ones are briefly described and further reading can be pursued by locating the complete references which appear at the end of this module.

The theories can be organized as **genetic aging theories, biochemical aging theories, physiological aging theories, and aging as sociopsychological development.** Most of the information which follows about current theories comes from the document titled <u>In Search of the Secrets of Aging</u> (1993), Department of Health and Human Resources (DHHS), NIH Pub. No. 93-2756.

Genetic aging theories

Genetic factors theories - Probably the most famous of the genetic factors theories is the one by Hayflick (1965). He observed that cells taken from old animals divided much less often than cells from younger animals and concluded from this that the species' life span is fixed and genetically determined at the level of the cell, specifically by the genetic code in DNA. Other investigators contributing to the DNA models were Comfort (1964; 1979), Watson (1969) and Orgel (1963), who varied the work to include RNA.

Longevity genes - More recent work about genes involves examining chromosomes contained in the cell's nucleus. For many years of a person's life, the pairs of chromosomes continue to divide to form new cells. As one ages, the dividing reaches a point where it stops. When this happens, DNA synthesis is blocked. This is known as **cell senescence**. Thus far, the research has been conducted on fruit flies and yeast, and 14 genes have been identified which seem to be related to this explantion of the aging process. Eventually, researchers hope to find human genes which demonstrate this same process.

Biochemical aging theories

Somatic mutation theory holds that exposure to low doses of radiation accelerates aging and shortens the life-span by mutating cells, thus rendering them unable to perform their normal functions. Genetic mutations occur and accumulate with increasing age, causing cells to deteriorate, eventually resulting in death. The theory was based on the observation that exposure of animals to low doses of radiation resulted in an increase in abnormal chromosomes which were similar to those found in old animals. Similar conclusions were also drawn from the observation that exposure to the sun accelerates aging in skin. (Curtis, 1966; Curtis & Miller, 1971; Failla, 1958). The theory explained little about the aging process because (1) the effect of radiation occurs mainly in dividing cells (such as the skin and red blood cells) while the effects of aging are seen mainly in cells that no longer divide (such as the nephrons of the kidney), (2) the number of cells that undergo mutation is too small to account for overall aging, and (3) most cells contain mechanisms for the repair of DNA.

Wear and tear theory assumes that human organisms are much like machines in the sense that continued use leads to worn out or defective parts, similar to the wearing out of parts in machinery (Sacher, 1966). However, this theory ignores the fact that increased use actually leads to improvements in some functions such as in muscle groups. Rather than wearing muscles out, exercise actually builds and strengthens muscles.

Deprivation theories attribute aging to inadequate delivery of essential nutrients and oxygen to cells of the body. The evidence for this was concluded from such effects as the localized death of brain cells following a stroke. Brain tissue and neurons died when deprived of oxygen. However, although there is localized damage due to oxygen deprivation in stroke cases, there is no evidence for systematic reduction of oxygen with advancing age.

Crosslinkage theory suggests that with aging, there is a chemical reaction that produces crosslinking of essential molecules in cells (which cannot be repaired), ranging from DNA within the nucleus to macromolecules such as protein. These crosslinked structures such as elastin and collagen (i.e., proteins in connective tissue) cause rigidity and decreased pliability in lungs, heart and supporting muscle, cartilage, and lining of blood vessels (Saxon & Etten, 1987). An accumulation of crosslinked proteins damages cells and tissues, slowing down bodily processes. The increased prevalence of osteoarthritis with age is an example of this theoretical perspective.

Accumulation theory emphasizes the build up of certain body substances over the years (such as lipofuscin or lipids) which ultimately interfere with cell efficiency to such an extent that the cell dies. A clinical example as evidence of this theory might be the accumulation of atherosclerotic plaques (Saxon & Etten, 1987).

Oxygen radicals - Some of the earliest work on this theory was done by Harman (1981) who proposed that most aging changes and degenerative diseases are due to free-radical damage. A free radical is a molecule with an unpaired, highly chemically reactive electron. An oxygen free radical is a byproduct of metabolism, produced as cells convert food and oxygen into energy. The free radical is extremely unstable and combines to form compounds which can damage proteins, cell membranes and nucleic acids, particularly DNA. Although the free radicals are rapidly destroyed by corrective mechanisms in the body including anti-oxidants such as vitamins C and E, and beta carotene, some damage still occurs which causes tissues and organs to break down (DHHS, 1993).

DNA repair - Throughout life, the DNA in cells is damaged by oxygen radicals, ultraviolet light and other toxic agents. This results in changes and/or losses of parts of the DNA which make up the genetic code. Researchers theorize that the DNA damage rises steadily over the lifespan, causing genes, proteins, and cells to function incorrectly, and tissues and organs to break down. However, it is also known that various enzyme systems in the cell exist to repair damaged DNA (DHHS, 1993).

Heat shock proteins - Cells in the body produce a type of protein called Heat Shock Proteins (HSPs), whenever the body is exposed to stressors, such as heat, toxic chemicals, and psychological strain. These seem to be protective against some of the aging processes. Scientists have found that the amount of HSPs produced is related to one's age. When animals are put under stress in experimental conditions, older ones produce *less* HSPs than younger ones. It is known that (1) HSPs work in cells to help break down and remove damaged proteins, (2) contribute to the making and transport of new proteins and (3) seem to be related to hormones released when one is stressed. However, how or why HSPs change as one ages is not yet understood (DHHS, 1993).

Hormones - It is known that the size and strength of muscles decrease as one ages. However, in a study where men aged 60 and older were given injections of recombinant human growth hormone (GH), it was found that (1) the hormone had reversed some signs of aging by increasing the size of muscles (that is muscle mass) and, (2) when the GH was stopped, muscle strength declined. GH is a synthetic version of the hormone that is produced in the pituitary gland, which has a major role growth and development of young people. Based on the study of GH, it seems that hormones have some role to play in the aging process. Other hormones currently under investigation include estrogen and testosterone (DHHS, 1993).

Glucose crosslinking - This is a more current and extensive version of the previously presented cross-linking model. In a process called non-enzymatic glycosylation, glucose molecules attach themselves to proteins forming a chemical reaction where proteins bind together or "crosslink". This interferes with their ability to carry out biological roles. The crosslinks called " advanced glycosylation end products " (AGEs), seem to make tissues less elastic. AGEs have been linked to changes seen typically in older persons including stiffening of collagen in connective tissue and hardening of arteries, changes in the eye, and decreased kidney filtration. Although the body has means of counteracting some AGE changes, AGEs increase steadily with age (DHHS, 1993). The changes which occur in older persons are also seen in younger people with diabetes who have high glucose levels. Therefore, diabetes has been studied as an accelerated model of aging. Glucose or blood sugar appears to be a factor in crosslinking that results in hardened tissue and deterioration (DHHS, 1993).

Physiological aging theories

Stress theory describes aging as the result of the additive effect, over time, of the effects of the stresses of living. Each time a stress occurs it leaves a residual impairment from which one does not fully recover. Eventually the cumulative stresses deplete one's body of needed reserves (Selye, 1966). The theory ignores the fact that, depending on how one learns to manage stress, the ability to handle stress and the side effects can actually be increased and improved.

Adaptation theory attributes aging to the failure of adaptive mechanisms (Blumenthal & Berns, 1964; Walford, 1969). For example, as one ages the antidiuretic hormone works less efficiently in preventing excess loss of body fluid through urination. There are many other ways in which the body's physiologic changes with age may evidence failure of adaptive mechanisms such as (1) the fact that receptor sites important to sugar metabolism are fewer, (2) breathing capacity diminishes and (3) immune response is thought to decrease.

Immune system role - Theories about **Immunity** and **Autoimmunity** go as far back as the researchers Blumenthal & Berns (1964), and Walford (1969). The theories are based on two observations: (1) that the functioning of the immune system decreases with age, as is evident in the decline in resistance to infectious disease in older adults, and (2) that there is an increase in autoimmune disease as one ages. The immune system includes the thymus, spleen, tonsils, bone marrow and lymphatic system. These produce many substances important to resisting infection including lymphocytes, antibodies, and interleukins (DHHS, 1993).

Lymphocytes are of two major types: B-cells and T-cells. B-cells (found in the bone marrow) secrete antibodies to overcome infections. T-cells are further divided into (1) cytotoxic T-cells and (2) helper T-cells. Cytotoxic T-cells attack infected or damaged cells directly; helper T-cells produce chemicals that assist other immune system substances to function. T-cells are formed in the thymus, which decreases in weight and ability to produce T-cells as one ages (DHHS, 1993).

It is known that the interleukins help regulate the immune system. Researchers have found that interleukin-6 rises with age. It is thought that this increase interferes with immune system response. Another observation has been that interleukin-2, which stimulates T-cell production thereby improving resistance to infection, declines as one ages (DHHS, 1993).

The decrease in immunological function may result in an increase in autoimmunological function. There is some evidence that there is an increase in autoantibodies in older people, which act to destroy normal cells (DHHS, 1993).

Calorie restriction - Research done on animals gives some support to the theory that less calories are better than more calories. Mice who were given 30 to 60% fewer calories than the comparison mice lived longer than the mice on higher calorie diets. Currently, the effect of dietary calories is being studied in other species and primates (DHHS, 1993).

Behavioural factors - Many different theories are being explored concerning behavioral factors. Some of the factors being investigated are the effects of dietary fat, calcium, vitamin D, and exercise and lifestyle changes (DHHS, 1993).

Aging as sociopsychological development

These theories have their evidence grounded in attitudinal, biographical, cognitive, and social context research. All of them describe aging in terms of psychological development and/or social interaction and developmental stages. The psychosocial processes are influenced by (1) patterns of change over adult years that appear in most individuals (such as the historical period, culture, personal development and self-esteem) and, (2) the idea that any theories which attempt to explain the aging process must consider these multiple influences in order to be meaningful. Although there are many such theories, only a few of the most well-known ones will be described.

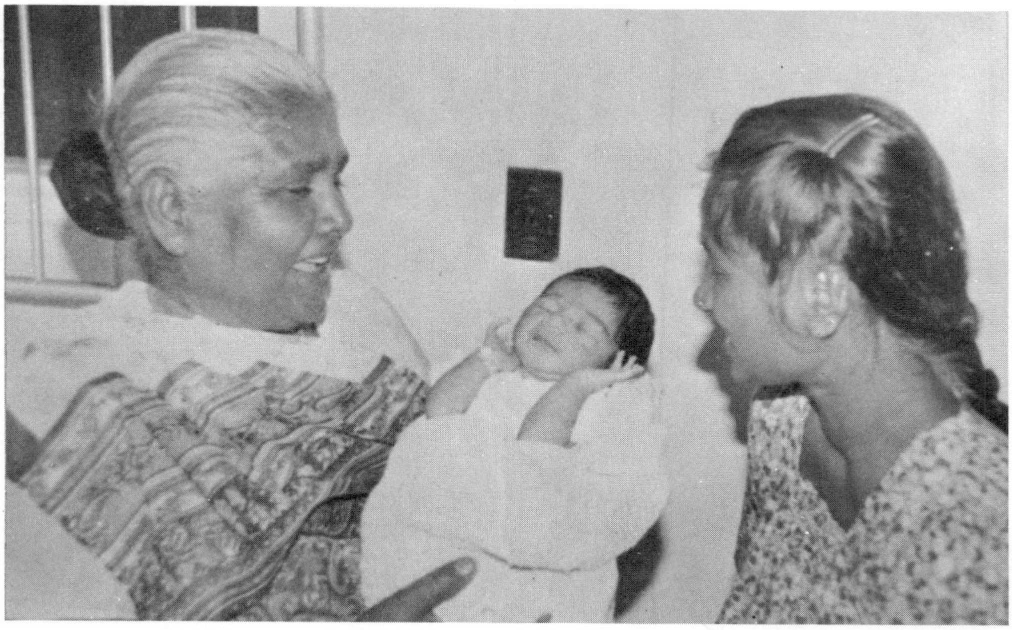

Photo courtesy of T. Miller

A role in caring for grandchildren adds meaning to life. This Fijian grandmother takes great satisfaction in teaching the mother, her daughter about baby care.

Personal meaning and purpose - This theory holds that all people need to have meaning in their lives. If meaning and purpose in life are lacking, hopelessness and depression set in, and eventually there is a loss of the will to go on living. Meaning and purpose in life are gradually discovered by each individual over the course of their life. By going beyond one's self-interests, being involved and committed to others, and accepting responsibilities, one gains greater meaning and purpose as one gets older. This suggests an emotionally healthy old age, while those who do not accomplish this have less satisfaction in their later years (Birren & Bengston, 1988).

Disengagement theory (Cumming & Henry, 1961) is the view that aging involves the withdrawal of older people from the roles characteristic of middle age. In other words, older people withdraw psychologically from previous forms of socialization, work and related activities. In this perspective, the situation is supposed to be mutually beneficial to older and younger persons alike. Older persons are considered to have a decreased capacity for involvement while at the same time, society needs to fit younger people into slots once occupied by the elderly.

Support for the theory was based on some observations of decreased number and frequency of social interactions as well as decreased emotional involvement in old age. The theory has been criticized on the grounds that (1) much withdrawal of older persons is not voluntary, (2) there is no consistent evidence for decrease of social/relational interaction, and (3) it is not seen in all cultural groups.

Activity theory - Activity theory has been described by Cavan (1962), Cavan et al. (1949), Havighurst & Albrecht (1953), and Lemon et al.(1972). It is in direct contrast to disengagement theory. It holds that the more active elderly persons are, the greater their satisfaction with life will be. The emphasis is on ongoing social interaction in the development of self concept in the elderly. Self concept is related to the roles one holds, but with old age comes loss of roles. In order to maintain a positive sense of self, the elderly must substitute new roles. Thus, well-being in late life results from increased activity in newly-acquired roles. It advocates continued activity and involvement in social activities.

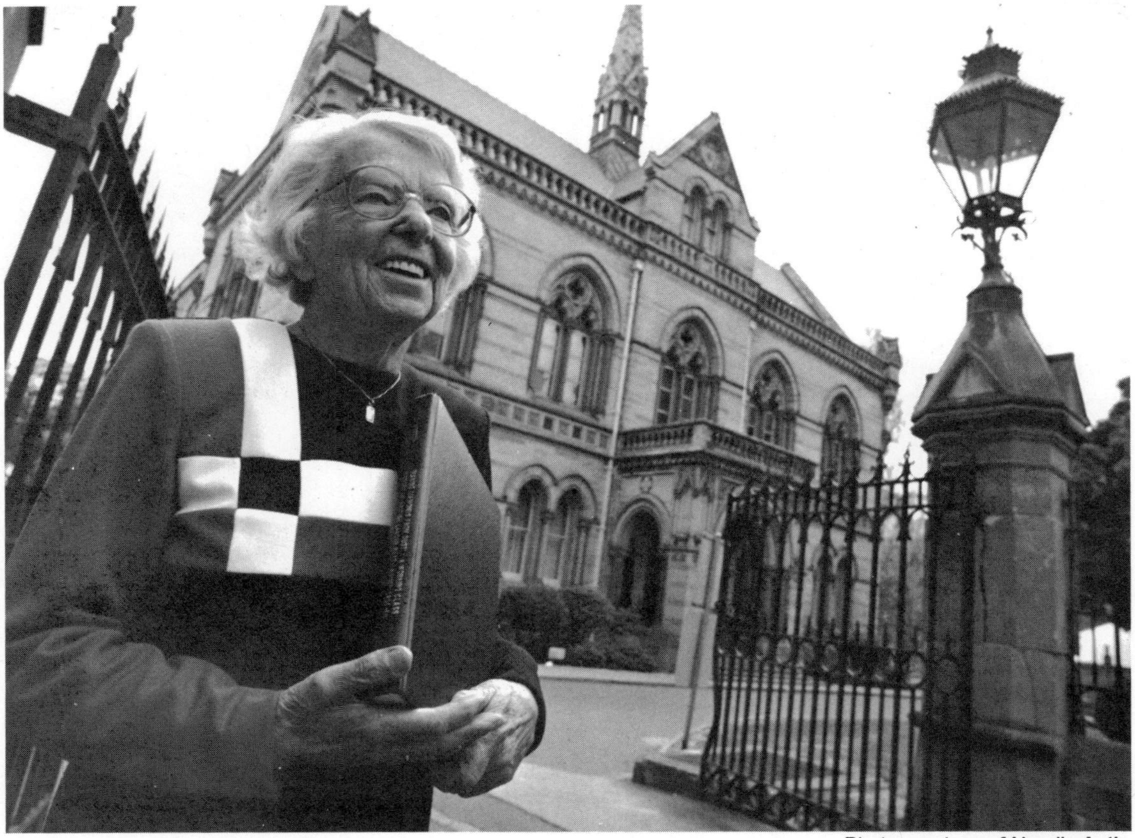

Photo courtesy of Narelle Autio

To maintain a positive sense of self, the elderly must acquire new roles. This 78-year old Australian lady has recently completed her 50,000-word Master of Arts thesis.

Support for this theory came from the observation that active older persons seemed to have greater feelings of contentment and life satisfaction than those who were inactive. Critics of the view argue that the theory (1) assumes all older people are alike in that they need and desire high levels of social activity (2) overlooks differences in the preference for types of activities, for example group activities as compared to individual activities as in reading and (3) suggests that *quantity* of relationships is more important than *quality*.

Continuity theory - The continuity theory holds that the critical factors in adjustment to old age are one's previously acquired coping abilities and the ability to maintain continuity with previous roles and activities (Havighurst,

1969). As one ages, there is an extension of the former self, and possibly an exaggeration. Knowledge of the individual's personality type is thought to be helpful in predicting their response to the aging process (Neugarten & Datan, 1973).

Functional capacity - Unlike genetic, biological, and physiological theories of aging, and also unlike sociopsychological explanations, description of the aging process according to function is more a belief system (based on practicalities) than an actual theory. The notion is that one's age is not a particularly important consideration in aging. The influential factor in framing older age concerns is how well persons function in regard to activities of daily living (ADLs) and instrumental activities of daily living (IADLs). Independence in ADLs and IADLs suggests healthy aging, while dependency indicates the presence of illness, disability and deterioration.

Exercise A

In this exercise, the instructor will review with you *the trends in aging for your respective country (or countries).* Following this you will draw a picture of yourself as you would be at 75 years of age. Share as a group what you are doing in the picture, where you are and other such things.

Short-answer exercise

1. Think about stereotyping of the elderly that occurs in advertisements, pictures and music. Jot down what you have observed or heard, why you suspect it may have originated, and a way in which you could help to change it.

2. Select one theory proposed to explain the aging process and apply it to a clinical health care situation.

Bibliography

Genetic, biochemical and physiological theories:

Birren, J.E. & Bengston, V.L. (Eds)(1988). Emergent theories of aging. New York: Springer.

Birren, J.E. & Schaie, K.W.(Eds.)(1977). Handbook of the psychology of aging. New York: Van Nostrand Reinhold.

Bjorksten, J. (1968). The cross linkage theory of aging. Journal of the American Geriatrics Society, 16: 408-427.

Brocklehurst, J.C. & Hawley, T. (1970). Geriatric medicine for students. London : Churchill Livingstone

Blumenthal, H.T. & Berns, A.W. (1964). Autoimmunity and aging. In B.L. Strehler (Ed). Advances in gerontological research, vol.1 (pp.289-342). New York: Academic Press.

Brookbank, J.W. (1990). The biology of aging. Philadelphia: Harper & Row.

Comfort, A. (1964). Ageing: The biology of senescence. New York: Holt, Rinehart & Winston.

Comfort, A. (3rd ed)(1979). Ageing: The biology of senescence. New York: Elsevier.

Curtis, H.J. (1966). Biological mechanisms of aging. Springfield, IL.: Charles C. Thomas.

Curtis, H.F. & Miller, K. (1971). Chromosome aberrations in lower cells of guinea pigs. Journal of Gerontology, 26: 292-293.

Department of Health & Human Services (1993). In search of the secrets of aging. National Institute on Aging, (NIH Publication No. 93-2756), Bethesda, MD, USA.

Failla, G. (1958). The aging process and carcinogenesis. Annals of the New York Academy of Sciences, 71: 1124-1135.

Finch, C.E. (1991). Longevity, senescence and the genome. Chicago: University of Chicago Press.

Hayflick, L. (1965). The limited in vitro lifetime of human diploid cell strains. Experimental Cellular Research, 37: 614-636.

Orgel, L.E. (1963). The maintenance of the accuracy of protein synthesis and its relevance to aging. Proceedings of the National Academy of Sciences of the United States of America, 49: 517-521.

Sacher, G.A. (1966). Abnutzungstheorie. In N.W. Shock (Ed). Perspectives in experimental gerontology, (pp.326-335). Springfield, Il.: Charles C. Thomas.

Saxon, S.V. & Etten, M.J.(1987). Physical change and aging: A guide for the helping professions (2nd Ed.). New York: Tiresias Press.

Selye, H. (1966). The future for aging research. In N.W. Shock (Ed). Perspectives in experimental gerontology, (pp.375-387). Springfield, Il.: Charles C. Thomas.

Walford, R.L. (1969). The immunologic theory of aging. Baltimore: Williams & Wilkins.

Warner, H., Butler, R.N., Sprott, R.L. & Schneider, E.L. (Eds.)(1987). Modern biological theories of aging. New York: Raven Press.

Watson, J.D. (1969). The double helix. New York: New American Library.

Sociopsychological development theories of aging

Birren, J.E. & Bengston, V.L. (Eds)(1988). Emergent theories of aging. New York: Springer.

Birren, J.E. & Schaie, K.W.(Eds.)(1977). Handbook of the psychology of aging. New York: Van Nostrand Reinhold.

Cavan, R.S. (1962). Self and role in adjustment during old age. In A. Rose (Ed). Human behavior and social processes. Boston: Houghton Mifflin.

Cumming, E. & Henry, W.E. (1961). Growing old: The process of disengagement. New York: Basic Books.

Havighurst, R.J. & Albrecht, R. (1953). Older people. New York: Longmans Green.

Havighurst, R.J., Neugarten, B.L., Munichs, J.M.A., & Thomae, H. (Eds). (1969). Adjustment to retirement: A cross-national study. Netherlands: Van Gorkum.

Lemon, B.W., Bengston, V.L. & Peterson, J.A. (1972). An exploration of the activity theory of aging: Activity types and life satisfaction among in-movers to a retirement community. Journal of Gerontology, 27: 511-523.

Neugarten, B. & Datan, N. (1973). Sociological perspectives on the life cycle. In P. Bates and K. Schaie (Eds). Lifespan developmental psychology: Personality and socialization. New York: Academic Press.

Background

Adelson, A. et al (1982). Behavioral ratings of health professionals' interactions with the geriatric patient. Gerontologist, 22(3): 277-281.

Austin, D.R. (1985). Attitudes toward old age: A hierarchical study. Gerontologist, 25(4): 431-434.

Binstock, R.H. (1983). . The aged as scapegoat. Gerontologist, 23(2): 136-142

Butler, R.N. & Lewis, M.I. (1977). Aging and mental health (2nd ed.). St. Louis: C.V. Mosby.

Davis, L.J. (1977). Attitudes toward old age and aging as shown by humor.

Gerontologist, 17(3): 220-225.

Erikson, E.H. (1963). Childhood and society. New York: Norton.

Kaplin, A., (Ed.) (1992). Health promotion and chronic illness: Discovering a new quality of health. Copenhagen: World Health Organization, European Series No. 44.

Kart, C.S.,& Metress, E.S. & Metress, J.F. (1978). Aging and health: biological and social perspectives. Menlo Park: Addison-Wesley.

Matteson, M.A. & McConnell, E.S. (1988). Gerontological nursing: Concepts and practice. Philadelphia: W.B. Saunders.

Palmore, E.B. (1990). Ageism: Negative and positive. New York: Springer.

Saxon, S.V. & Etten, M.J. (1987). Physical change and aging: A Guide for the Helping Professions (2nd ed.) New York : Tiresias Press.

Senses

MODULE 2 - *THE SENSES*

Objectives

On completion of this module, the student should be able to:

1. describe the normal age-related changes which occur in the senses and the implications of these:

   - skin
   - vision
   - hearing
   - taste
   - smell
   - touch, sensation and balance;

2. screen for normal age-related sensory decrements;

   - assess all senses
   - identify and prioritize alterations
   - develop care plans including goals and interventions for education and safety
   - propose ways of evaluating the effectiveness of the care plan;

3. identify common health problems, (that is deviations from expected age-related changes in the senses); and

4. develop care plans (with goals and interventions) for common problems and ways of evaluating the effectiveness.

Introduction

Connective tissue consists of cells and extracellular fibres embedded in an amorphous ground material or matrix. Connective tissue protects, supports, and binds organs together, acts as a shock absorber, and allows expansion and contraction of tissue. In the extracellular material, there are three types of fibres. Two of the most important of these in terms of aging are collagen and elastin.

Collagen is a ropelike protein fibre which provides strength and resists stretching. ***Elastin*** is a rubberband type fibre which gives tissue its elastic qualities. The fibres are loosely intertwined and work together to give the human body a smooth, easy movement.

As one ages, collagen and elastin crosslink to form strong dense bonds rather than remaining loosely intertwined. The collagen becomes stiff and the elastin becomes calcified and loses its elasticity.

> Connective tissue accounts for almost one-third of the protein in the body, so changes in the collagen and elastin greatly affect the functioning of nearly all body systems. Among the areas affected are *the senses and muscles which support the sensory organs, the musculoskeletal system including cartilage, and the cardiovascular, urinary and respiratory systems.*

Normal age-related changes in the senses

Skin

The skin is the largest organ of sense and the first line of defence for the body. In the aging skin, there are changes in the collagen and elastin as just described, plus decreased vascularity, increased capillary fragility, reduction and relocation of subcutaneous fat, and change in pigment. Nails on the hands and feet become tough and brittle.

Sweat and oil glands perform less effectively and secrete less lubrication. This tends to make the skin dry.

On some parts of the body, pigmentation may increase. For example, in fair-skinned people, brown pigmented spots typically appear on the hands. These are called liver or age spots, and are caused by the build up of lipofuscin which gives rise to the dark pigment. The medical term for these spots is **lentigo senilis**.

In hair, the pigment decreases, thereby causing it to gray. Gray hair is simply hair that has lost its colour or pigment. In addition , the hair follicles atrophy, and by about age 50, as much as one-third of the follicles may be lost . The loss may continue in later years at the rate of about 1% per year. Changes in hormones may create facial hair in women and hair loss in both men and women.

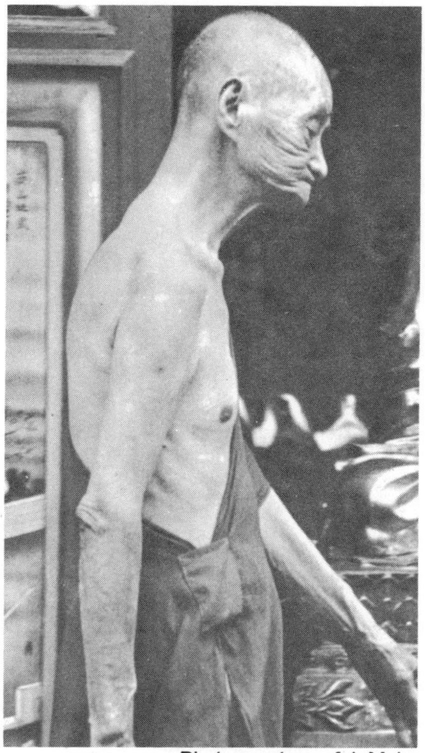

Photo courtesy of J. Mohr

Skin of older people loses tone, becomes wrinkled, thinner and more fragile, and is more susceptible to cuts and bruises.

As a result, the skin of older people loses turgor (that is tone), becomes wrinkled, thinner and more fragile, and is more susceptible to cuts and bruises. The distribution of subcutaneous (SQ) fat changes. It decreases on the face, neck, arms, hands, legs and feet, and increases on the hips, abdomen, organs and muscles. Bony prominences are therefore less padded and appear more noticeable.

IMPLICATIONS AND RECOMMENDATIONS

The skin of older people is much more susceptible to injury even from minor bumps and scrapes. Complaints of pruritus (i.e., itching) are common, and in people with lighter skin tone, the incidence of skin cancer is increased. If older people are immobilized for any length of time, pressure sores are especially likely. One must (1) be very gentle in handling and holding onto them, (2) make sure certain objects which might cause injury aren't sticking out in their environment, (3) use soaps and bathing products which keep the skin as moist as possible, and (4) use lotions as needed and protective garments when in the sun. Because of the loss of body fat, older people tend to be more susceptible to cold, even at mildly chilly temperatures. They should be kept in appropriately warm clothing.

NOTE: Many physiological changes in older adults make them more likely to suffer low body temperatures **(hypothermia)** due to cold and/or **dehydration** from excessive heat.

Vision

The appearance of the eye changes. The pigment in the iris becomes paler and there is a deposit of lipid that forms a whitish gray ring at the outer edge of the iris. It is usually quite obvious and it forms a halo around the iris. This circle is called **arcus senilis**.

Weakening of the elasticity of ocular muscles and loss of fat in tissue around the eye may cause the eyelid to droop in very old people. This is called **senile ptosis**. There is also decreased production of tears.

Within the structure of the eye, the pupil becomes smaller and less light enters due to narrowing of the opening. The lens changes from clear to yellow, called the **"Yellow Filter Effect"** (Saxon & Etten, 1987) and this too reduces the amount of light that reaches the eye. Together, the smaller pupil size and the yellowing of the lens may result in as much as 50% less light entering the retina.

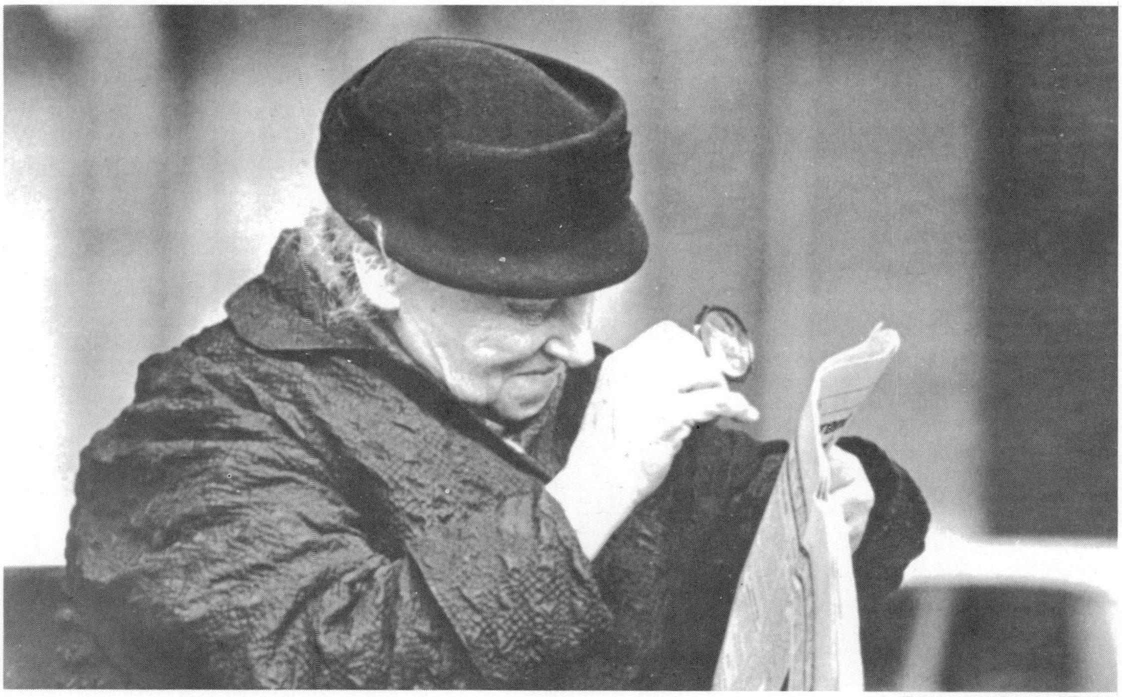

Photo courtesy of Zafar

Eyes of older people have changed. They need more light to see adequately.Care should be taken to promote a safe environment in order to prevent injury.

By age 40, the lens of the eye becomes less pliable and the ciliary muscles which hold the lens in place lose tone. As a result, the eyes of older people are less able to adjust between near and far vision. The far-sightedness (that is the inability to read things which are close at hand) associated with aging is termed **presbyopia**. There is no exercise or medication that will reverse this process. Reading glasses or bifocals are necessary to help the eye focus.

As a result of changes in the eye, older persons:

- are less able to see small objects and details,
- are less able to shift their sight quickly from near to far vision and vice versa,
- have trouble with depth perception,
- are extremely sensitive to glare,
- are bothered more by eye irritation, and
- do not see all colours equally well. Red, orange and yellow tones are seen better than blue, green and purple shades.

IMPLICATIONS AND RECOMMENDATIONS

Older persons need more light in order to see adequately. This is true for reading as well as for seeing to get about safely in their environment. Since they have difficulty with depth perception and glare, doors should never be left partially open, as this poses problems in perception and makes doors a likely target for injury. Stairs are also a problem in perceived depth, as are floors and walls which are all of the same colour. Some forms of artificial lighting (such as fluorescent), also cause problems for glare and depth perception. Keep objects in their environment in the same place so that they know exactly where things are located. Remove scatter rugs and have them wear practical shoes.

Even prior to formal assessment, *behaviour* may give clues about visual problems. For example, frequent falls, wearing mismatched clothes or wearing clothes inside-out can be clues that age-related visual decrements exist. Simple tests of vision can be done with the use of pocket size Snellen charts (A copy is on the following page). If a person cannot read, pictures of objects of varying sizes may work better in assessments than the lettered Snellen chart. Uncompensated visual problems can make older people less independent.

Hearing

Subtle changes in hearing begin in the forties. Over time, the eardrum and membrane over the oval window thicken and become more rigid. Ear wax (cerumen) also thickens and becomes more difficult to dissolve. There is gradual atrophy and degeneration of hair cells (cilia) and decreased blood supply to the cochlea which result in reduced discrimination, especially to consonants, *trills* (e.g., rr sounds) and *sibilants* (e.g., s z sh zh sounds).

For example in regard to *sibilants* (g f s z t sh ch sl th) which are difficult to hear:

The question: "Oh, do you like that?" might be heard as "Oh, do you like fat?" because the TH sounds like F.

The question: "Is your chair comfortable?" might be heard as "Is your hair comfortable?" because the CH sound gets lost.

NOTE: Depending on the country and language spoken, these sounds may or may not pose a great deal of trouble. Other hearing difficulties may be more important. In the Japanese language for example, the *range of voice* and *similarity in modulation and loudness* create more difficulty in hearing for elders than the distinction of consonants.

Presbycusis is loss of hearing which is common in older persons. High frequency sounds are affected first with progression to lower frequency sounds. Men are affected a little more than women. Approximately 30% of people over 65 have significant hearing impairment.

IMPLICATIONS AND RECOMMENDATIONS

Uncompensated hearing decrements can make older people appear to be mentally impaired and/or withdrawn when they are not. Inadequate hearing can result in lack of understanding and the older person's inappropriate response or expression may be mistakenly interpreted as confusion or problems with mental status. Hearing loss can also interfere with socialization. If listening becomes too much of an effort or too embarrassing, older persons may eventually give up trying to hear what is being said, and talk and participate less.

The following behaviour may suggest high frequency hearing loss associated with aging:

- the older person tends to shout and/or others tend to speak very loudly to them;
- the older person often requests to have things repeated;
- the older person talks little, appears not to participate, or appears to ignore what is going on when in a group of people; and
- the older person becomes suspicious that things are being said about them.

In addition to these observations, there are several simple tests which can give one some idea of the older person's hearing ability. One of them involves standing approximately three feet behind the older person. Using a normal speaking tone, state the following words one by one and have the older person repeat them after you.

smart spare off with that thin will cat room all jaw does

Notice which words are difficult to the older person to hear. If the older person cannot repeat many of the words, *do the exercise again facing them directly* and using good light. Be sure to leave enough time between words so that they don't all run together. (Source: Shore, [1978] in Wolanin and Philipps, 1981).

If the older person cannot hear and repeat the words without you facing them, but *can do* the exercise while *facing you*, this may mean that the hearing loss is at least partially compensated by lip reading. If the older person cannot perform well even face-to-face, this may be evidence of more pronounced hearing loss, or an indication that visual limitations prevent lip reading.

Ear wax is frequently a cause of, or at least aggravates, hearing difficulties, therefore this should be the first thing checked. Cleaning the ear is usually preceded by insertion of drops to loosen the cerumen.

Sometimes a hearing aid can be helpful. However, be sure that the older person and the family know how to (1) insert the appliance, (2) turn it on and off properly, (3) know the battery type and where to get more, and (4) know how to test and replace the batteries. Whenever communicating with the older person, speak slowly, facing the person, and lower the pitch of your voice. If you raise your voice, this only creates more high frequency sounds and these are the ones most difficult to hear. Keeping the voice low is more helpful. It is important to eliminate or at least reduce environmental noise. In group situations, try to avoid having several conversations going on at once. When interviewing older persons, be certain to conduct the meeting in the quietest place possible, reinforcing verbal and auditory messages with written communication.

Taste and smell

Taste receptors are located primarily in taste buds of the tongue. With age, the number of taste buds diminishes. The remaining buds have a higher threshold and require stronger stimulation to activate them. It is uncertain whether taste and smell decline enough with age to interfere with the enjoyment of eating. It takes more flavour or spice to stimulate taste, but there are more than tastebuds to provide stimulation. The *perception* of how things taste may be impaired by age-related changes in smell. Older persons may be observed to add several spoonfuls of sugar to their coffee or tea. This is probably not done because they suddenly get a sweet-tooth with age, but more likely because it takes more sugar for them to notice the sweet taste. The same excess can happen in the use of salt and this can pose many difficulties. In addition to the changes in the taste buds, there is

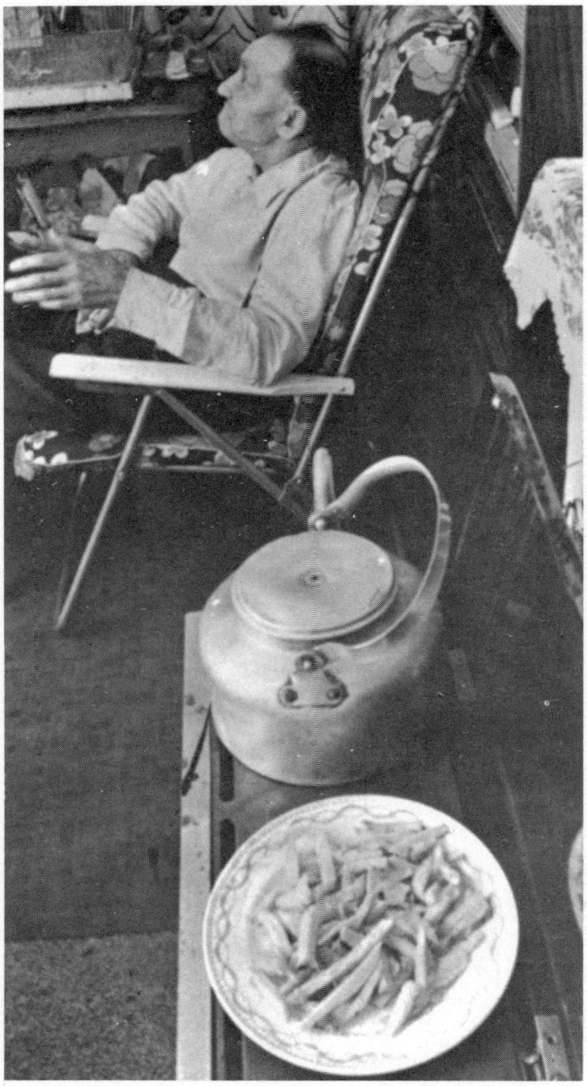

Photo courtesy of Zafar

With age the number of taste buds diminishes. Make food appealing and assess regularly the nutritional status of the elderly.

decreased salivary secretion. Poor dental hygiene, absence of teeth, and/or poorly fitting dentures also can alter the sensation of taste.

Taste and smell go hand in hand. Receptors for smell are located in the lining of nasal passages and the number of nerve fibres decreases with age.

IMPLICATIONS AND RECOMMENDATIONS

The combined effects of changes in taste and smell can:

- make food taste less appealing, thereby reducing food intake and impairing nutritional status;
- conflict with recommended dietary limitations, for instance moderate use of salt and sugar, since reasonable use is hard to taste; and
- interfere with the ability of smell and taste to protect the elderly from harm. For example, if older persons cannot smell smoke, they may

be unaware of a fire hazard. If spoiled foods cannot be detected, spoiled food products may be eaten.

Evaluation of smell and taste are frequently overlooked in older people. Both can be done easily. To check smell, have the older person close their eyes while you place various pungent substances under their nose, and ask them to identify the substances. Peanut butter, cloves, citrus and other fruits, tea, coffee, and other strong scents are good substances to use. To assess taste, have the person keep their eyes closed and use strongly flavoured substances such as sugar, salt, mint, and lemon juice on the tongue. Be certain to offer some water in between tastes to clear the taste buds of the previous substance.

Most interventions for age-related decrements in taste and smell involve education of the older person and the family about the changes in these senses, and the possible dangers to safety which may be associated with them. For example, rather than smelling foods to determine whether they are spoiled, put a date on the container, or for things such as milk, read the date on the label.

NOTE: *Reading dates on labels can be very difficult for older persons because the print is usually very small.*

If excessive use of salt or sugar poses a problem in dietary management, the use of spices (such as garlic, curry) may be suggested to enhance the flavour of foods. In countries such as Japan, it may be preferable to use salt-reduced and low-calorie foods. Adjustment of dentures and frequent mouth care are also recommended.

Touch and vestibular and kinesthetic senses

The sense of touch is associated with the ability to feel differences in temperature, the ability to feel pressure, the perception of pain, proprioception or position sense, crude and fine touch sense, and localization sense (Wolanin & Phillips, 1981). There is some evidence that older persons may not react or feel heat, cold, and pain as well as younger persons. Body sway increases with age and alters equilibrium and balance.

IMPLICATIONS AND RECOMMENDATIONS

Assessment of touch can be performed with simple materials. The skin can be brushed with cotton, the point of a pin and coarse materials and fabrics to get some idea of the older person's sense of tactile response.

The *primary concern* with change in this sensory domain is for *safety*.

Older persons may not realize when water is too hot. One must be very careful that shower or tub water does not cause scalding (1st degree burns).

Older persons should be instructed to walk using a wide gait in order to give them a better base of support and to compensate for sway. Holding onto someone or holding onto stable objects, such as canes or walkers, is also important. It is advisable for the elderly to avoid climbing up onto chairs and stepstools and using ladders.

NOTE: *Try to anticipate their needs and get things they need ahead of time.*

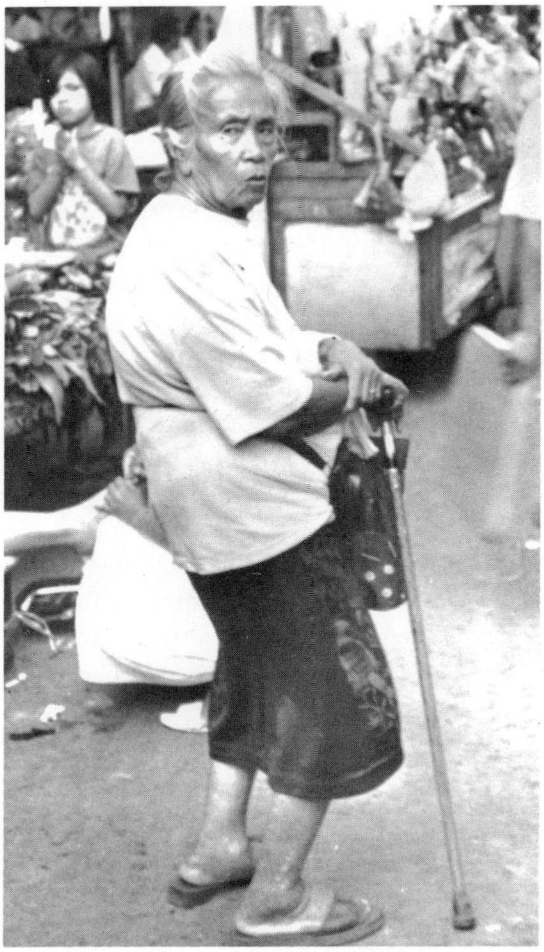

Photo courtesy of T. Miller

Body sway increases with age and alters equilibrium and balance. To prevent falls, instruct older people to walk using a wider gait and to hold something, such as a cane, to stabilize themselves.

SUMMARY

Sensory alterations can result in:

- sensory deprivation or sensory limitation below what is needed for independent functioning;
- sensory overload which may overwhelm elders and also prevent effective functioning; or sensory distortion that interferes with the older person's ability to understand and correctly interpret clues in the environment (Wolanin & Phillips, 1981).

If these results occur, dysfunctional behavioural changes may follow including confusion, avoidance of needed social interactions, isolation, sleep disturbances, loss of appetite, irritability and depression. There are also many safety problems which can arise.

Alteration in senses which are not a normal part of the aging process but which are frequently problems

Skin

Herpes zoster, also known as shingles, is an acute viral infection which may afflict older people. It is caused by herpesvirus *varicellae* which also causes chicken pox in children. Symptoms begin with burning pain along a nerve pathway, followed by a papular rash of three to four days, then vesicular and pustular eruptions, and finally crusting. Herpes zoster is most often located in the thoracic or lumbosacral areas and on the face and neck.

The pain can be very severe during the active course of the disease and chronic pain may persist at the site for many years (called post-herpetic neuralgia).

Treatment is directed towards relief of pain and prevention of infection. Good hygiene is critical and gentle handling of the affected parts, along with medications as ordered.

Dermatitis in the elderly is a special concern because the skin irritation is an additional problem to the already dry skin and is more resistant to treatment. The most common types in people over 50 years of age are allergic eczematous contact dermatitis, allergic drug reactions and allergic urticaria (hives) [Chin, 1971]. Treatment is directed to the underlying cause, management of itching, and prevention of infection.

> Decubitus ulcers (for those who remain in bed) and stasis ulcers (from poor venous return) are common in older persons. They require extensive treatment which varies depending on the degree of the ulcer and the cause.

Eyes

Cataracts are the clouding of the normally clear lens of the eye. This condition decreases visual function and can interfere with the older person's ability to live and function independently.

Cataracts usually develop in both eyes in persons over 50 and are present to some extent in most persons over 70 years of age. Multiple factors are supposed to contribute to their development such as family history, nutritional problems, severe diarrhoea episodes, ultraviolet-B radiation, diabetes, drugs, smoking, low antioxidant vitamin status, medications such as steroids, previous eye surgery, and alcohol use.

Cataract formation is characterized by (painless) blurring, and increasing but gradual loss of vision, increased sensitivity to glare or light, and general darkening of vision. Signs and symptoms include (1) need for frequent eyeglass prescription changes, (2) needing brighter light to read, (3) poor night vision, and (4) fading or yellowing of colours. When cataracts cause major difficulties with daily routines, then surgery is the treatment of choice. After the lens is removed, it is necessary to give the eye some other form of focusing ability. This is done in one of three ways: (1) surgical implantation of an intraocular lens; (2) use of eyeglasses; or (3) use of contact lenses.

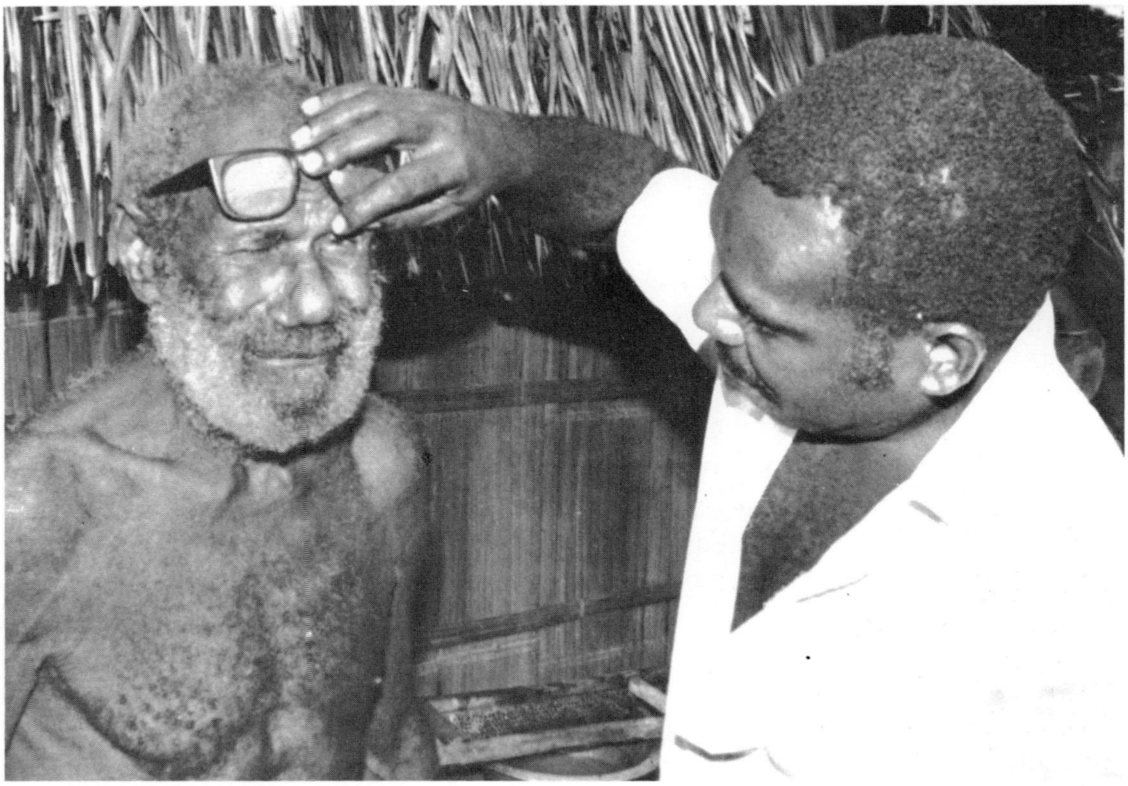

Photo courtesy of T. Miller

Cataracts decrease visual function. A Vanuatu nurse practitioner examines this village elderly and arranges for him to have surgical treatment by the mobile medical team.

Glaucoma is a condition in which there is increased intraocular pressure due to a defect in the outflow of aqueous humour. In untreated cases, the optic nerve (the nerve of sight) becomes damaged, usually because the fluid pressure inside the eye remains too high. Loss of vision from glaucoma can be prevented if the disease is detected and treated before noticeable damage occurs to the optic nerve. *More than any other eye condition, glaucoma needs to be detected early.* Glaucoma steals vision without any noticeable symptoms and many older people are not aware that they have the problem. Of the various types of glaucoma the following two are most often seen in older persons:

- **Open angle or chronic glaucoma** in which there is loss of peripheral vision late in the disease. This is the most common type of glaucoma in older people. Vision loss usually begins with deteriorating side vision, also known as "tunnel vision". It can happen so gradually and painlessly that the older person is unaware of any trouble until the optic nerve is already badly damaged. The diagnosis is made by measurement of intraocular pressure using specialized equipment.

- **Narrow angle glaucoma** occurs when there is a sudden blocking of the drainage angle of the eye. Extreme pain, coloured halos around lights, headaches, nausea and vomiting, and blurred vision are *symptoms* of this type of glaucoma. If this condition is not attended to urgently, blindness results.

Older persons should be screened for glaucoma and those with any known history of the disease need periodic examinations.

Degeneration of the macula increases with age and frequently occurs in both eyes. The macula, which is located in the retina, contains the fovea or central focusing point for the eye. The fovea processes the sharp central vision used for reading and other small or fine tasks. When the macula loses its ability to function fully, vision becomes blurred, and there is darkness or sometimes an empty area in the center of vision. Words on a page appear blurred so reading is difficult, and threading a needle may be impossible.

With age, the function of the macula is reduced due to decreased blood supply and tissue atrophy, and disease and nutritional factors can also contribute to macular deterioration.

In early stages there is moderate loss of vision, but if not properly diagnosed and monitored, it can progress to major central vision loss. Diagnosis is made by an opthalmoscope, and treatment is often with laser.

Diabetic retinopathy is the most common eye complication of diabetes mellitus. The retinal blood vessels (the light sensing nerve layer) at the back of the eye deteriorate. The condition is characterized by weakened retinal capillaries which may leak blood or fluid into the vitreous humor, causing scarring and/or retinal detachment. Vision may become blurred, distorted or partially blocked. If untreated, this condition can lead to detachment of the retina and blindness. Not all people with diabetes develop retinopathy, but the longer a person has diabetes, the greater the chance of developing this condition.

The major symptom is central vision impairment, although complete blindness is rare, and the goal of treatment is to retard visual impairment. Until recently, very little could be done to stop diabetic retinal changes. Now laser treatment is used to seal leaking blood vessels and reduce the chance of vision loss.

The term Laser stands for Light Amplification by Stimulated Emission of Radiation. An electric current is passed through a tube containing a gas (for example argon, krypton). Energy is produced and the laser emits a narrow uniform light beam which, when focused through a microscope, produces (1) heat coagulation, (2) cutting, or (3) dissolving of tissue. The advantages of Laser treatment include that there is less risk for infection than surgical procedures, it is fairly painless, and can be done without admitting the older person for long hospital stays.

Exercise A

The first step in obtaining accurate information about the elderly is to gain their trust and confidence. This section contains information and exercises to help you accomplish this. In this exercise, students will practice interviewing one another. Role-play with one student taking the part of the older person and the other taking the part of the health care worker. Do this in front of the entire group of students and analyse how well (and how completely) the interview was done. Read all the points which follow before you begin.

Older people may be fearful or uncomfortable when talking to health care workers whom they do not know well. In order to help put them at ease and provide important information about themselves, some communication strategies can be helpful. Techniques that encourage a good exchange include (1) listening well (that is active listening); (2) empathizing (which is showing that you understand the feelings of the person while at the same time remaining objective); and (3) using verbal and non-verbal approaches which centre upon open-ended and directed questioning.

Verbal techniques you will wish to emphasize include:

Clarification:	"I'm not clear about what you just said. Please explain in more detail."
Elaboration:	"Yes, please go on". "In addition to listening to music, how else do you spend your free time?"
Silence:	(older person) "It upset me quite a bit." (health care worker sits quietly).
Repeating:	(older person) "It upset me quite a bit." (health care worker) "Upset?"
Confirming or Acknowledging:	(health care worker) "Yes, I understand what you mean."
Summarization:	"Before we go on, let me summarize what you've told me so far."
Reflection:	(health care worker) "When you mentioned your children just now, you looked very proud."
Reassurance:	"It's alright to feel sad about the loss of your husband."

Verbal approaches which need to be avoided are ones which:

Limit the choice of response:	"What was your occupation?"
Use an either/or statement:	"Did you grow up in a rural or urban area?"

Interpret what the older person is telling you: "It sounds as if you are quite content with your lifestyle."

Evaluate and make a judgement: "That sounds reasonable to me."

In addition to the spoken words, non-verbal communication is very important and often gives a great deal of assessment data. Be alert to:

1. body language (posture, facial expressions, eye contact);
2. physical appearance (weakness or paralysis, arthritis) which may give clues about pain or functional limitations; and
3. physical distance and physical contact (which may tell you something about closeness, cultural perspective, fear and so on).

Exercise B

As a result of normal age-related changes in the eyes, older people have difficulty seeing many things and their vision may be distorted. Develop a plan of care including goals, interventions and means of evaluating the effectiveness for three problems with activities of daily living (ADLs) which you expect they might experience. The next few pages contain information on care planning and nursing diagnoses. Share the plans of care with the group.

Short-answer exercise

1. Briefly describe the changes in the eye. What behaviour in the older person gives clues that visual problems exist?

2. What is the primary concern for the elderly that results from age-related changes in the sense of <u>touch</u>?

Suggested field experience for assessment of practical skills

Students can be given the opportunity to *assess the senses* for an older adult. The clinical setting is arranged and materials be provided to students by the facilitator. The students should take notes on their findings and impressions. They should also identify and prioritize alterations in the senses, develop a care plan *for at least one activity of daily living which is affected by the sensory change*, including interventions for education and safety, and explain how the effectiveness of the plan is to be evaluated. The next page contains an example of a guideline to help them with this exercise. The pages following the guidelines have additional information on care planning and nursing diagnoses.

INSTRUCTORS PLEASE NOTE: A hand-held, pocket Snellen Chart (to assess distance vision) is in the back of this manual. You will need to provide additional ones to the students.

GUIDELINES
Senses and development of a plan of care
(EXAMPLE)

Area to be assessed	Supplies needed/technique	Normal change YES/NO	Compen-sated change YES/NO	Describe
		(NA=not applicable)		
SKIN:				
turgor	pinch the skin lightly and elevate	Y	Y	drinks adequate fluid
dryness	observe and feel	Y	Y	uses lotion
lentigo senilis	observe	N	NA	dark complexion
hand nails	observe	Y	NA	
toe nails	observe	Y	N	needs a podiatrist, nails thick, tough and overgrown
hair	observe	NA		uses hair dye
REMARKS: There are many bruises on the forearms and lower legs				
EYES:				
arcus senilis	observe	Y	NA	
ability to see print at a distance	hand-held pocket Snellen Chart	Y	Y	wears glasses for distance
abiity to distinguish colours	have objects of different colours or point to objects which are blue, green, orange, yellow and red	Y		could tell red and yellow better than blue

Planning care for the older person

Written plans aid communication among health care workers, family members and the older person. The plan includes the *problems* which have been identified, the *goals* to be achieved, the *interventions* to achieve the goals and *evaluation* of the degree to which goals have been achieved at any particular point in time. In order to develop a good and realistic plan, health care workers must systematically engage in problem-solving together with the older person, his or her family members, and collaborating health disciplines as appropriate.

THE PLAN (An example of a form is on page 20 of this module)

The plan should include the following:

1. Problems (actual and potential);
2. Goals;
3. Health care interventions; and
4. Evaluation (how well have goals been achieved).

Assessment and identification of problems

Assessment data should be recorded on a form organized in a manner that permits efficient data collection, such as the example given on page 20. In addition to going through all the systems (in this exercise it is the senses), consider the following:

1. What is usual for this older person?
2. What findings are not usual?
3. Does the person's usual pattern pose an actual problem or a potential problem?
4. What health promotion teaching is needed?

The assessment process concludes with the formulation of the problems, ideally in nursing diagnosis terminology. A *list of nursing diagnoses* is on page 21 of this module. Nursing diagnoses should be prioritized so that the most important and/or immediate problems receive attention first. Proceed as follows:

1. Identify the actual or potential problem(s) as stated on the list of nursing diagnoses.
2. Use your clinical judgement to put the problems in priority order. Ones that are high on the list may be so because they are most important to restoring function, they are an immediate safety concern, they are easiest to resolve and so on. List the problems in nursing

diagnosis terms in order of priority by numbering them from #1, meaning the highest priority, onwards.

Health care goals and evaluation

Goals should be measurable and written in terms of the older person's achievement. Several examples are provided which show the difference between well-written and poorly-written goals.

Example 1

POOR: The client will be provided instruction about good nutrition.

ANALYSIS: This is written in terms of the health care worker rather than in terms of the older person.

BETTER: The client will demonstrate knowledge about good nutrition by planning meals OR; The client will be able to plan meals using foods in recommended amounts from the four food groups.

Example 2

POOR: The client will be provided safety in their environment.

ANALYSIS: This is not measurable. There will be no way to evaluate whether the environment was made safe or not. It is also written in terms of the health care worker rather than in terms of the older person.

BETTER: The client will be safe in their environment as indicated by the absence of falls and other injuries.

Example 3

POOR: The client's vision will improve.

ANALYSIS: This is not specific enough to allow good evaluation.

BETTER: The client will be able to read fine print (that is, regular size reading materials)

Interventions

In deciding what interventions to use, be creative and realistic. The following are a few examples:

Example 1

GOAL: The client will demonstrate knowledge about good nutrition by planning meals.

INTERVENTIONS:
1. Review a food shopping list with the person.
2. Review the cost of foods and suggest what food equivalents might be less expensive.
3. Accompany the person to buy foods.
4. Have the person create a five-day meal plan for all meals.
5. Cut out pictures from newspapers or magazines to help illustrate.

Example 2

GOAL: The client will be safe in their environment as indicated by the absence of falls and other injuries.

INTERVENTIONS:
1. Ask the family to remove scattered rugs, loose floor mats, or boards.
2. Discuss safety aspects of the environment with the family and older person.
3. Have the family paint a bright yellow stripe on the stair outside the front door so the client can see where the step ends more easily.
4. Help the family get additional lights for the living room.
5. If cooking with charcoal, check that the surrounding area will not catch fire, such as the bed.

Example 3

GOAL: The client will be able to read fine print (that is, regular size reading materials)

INTERVENTIONS:
1. Make an appointment for an eye exam.
2. Arrange transportation to the clinic.
3. Make arrangements to pick up the eye glasses in 10 days.
4. Assess the older person's reading with the new glasses and again in about one week, in order to give some adjustment time.
5. Interview client and family to determine whether the older person is reading more or can see better to walk with the glasses.

REMEMBER: Develop the plan in collaboration with other members of the health care team as appropriate, the older person and family members. ***The best plan is useless if people aren't motivated to achieve it.*** Leave a copy of the plan with the older person's family.

PLAN OF CARE

Date onset	Nursing diagnosis health problems	Health care goals	Interventions	Date achieved

Evaluation notes:

Nursing Diagnosis Categories

(Based on L.J. Carpenito, Handbook of Nursing Diagnosis, 1989-90)

1. **Respiratory**
   Airway clearance, ineffective
   Breathing pattern, ineffective
   Gas exchange, impaired

2. **Circulatory**
   Cardiac output, alteration in
   Tissue perfusion, alteration (specify)

3. **Integumentary**
   Skin integrity impaired, actual
   Skin integrity impaired, potential for

4. **Nutritional metabolic**
   Fluid volume, alteration, excess
   Fluid volume deficit, actual (Regular failure)
   Fluid volume deficit, active loss
   Fluid volume deficit, potential
   Nutrition alteration, less than required
   Nutrition alteration, more than required
   Oral mucous membranes, altered
   Swallowing, impaired

5. **Elimination**
   Bowel elimination, alteration in (constipation)
   Bowel elimination, alteration in (diarrhoea)
   Bowel elimination, alteration in (incontinence)
   Urinary incontinence, functional
   Urinary incontinence, overflow
   Urinary incontinence, stress
   Urinary incontinence, urge
   Urinary retention, acute/chronic

6. **Muscular-skeletal**
   Activity intolerance
   Activity intolerance, potential for
   Mobility, impaired physical

7. **Coping and self-perception, self-concept**
   Adjustment, impaired
   Anxiety, (specify)
   Coping, ineffective individual
   Decisional conflict, (specify)
   Fear
   Grieving, anticipatory
   Grieving, dysfunctional
   Hopelessness
   Powerlessness
   Self-concept, disturbance in body image
   Spiritual distress
   Violence, potential for

8. **Cognitive-perceptive**
   Comfort, alteration, pain, acute
   Comfort, alteration, pain, chronic
   Communication, impaired, verbal
   Sensory perceptual alteration (specify), visual, auditory, kinesthetic, taste, touch, smell
   Thought processes, alteration
   Inappropriate behaviour (specify), aggressive, assaultive, wandering, others

9. **Sleep-rest**
   Sleep pattern disturbance

10. **Role-relationship**
    Coping, family, potential for growth
    Coping, ineffective family
    Diversionary activity, deficit
    Family process alteration
    Self concept, disturbance in role
    Social interaction, impaired
    Social isolation

11. **Self-care**
    Self-care deficit (specify), feeding, bathing, dressing, toileting
    Health maintenance alteration
    Home maintenance management, impaired
    Knowledge deficit (specify)
    Learning need (specify)
    Compliance, alteration in

12. **Potential for injury**
    Body temperature, potential alteration
    Hyperthermia
    Hypothermia
    Injury, potential for
    Infection, potential for

Bibliography

Senses

Aston, T. (June 1990). Empowering Visually Impaired People to Access their Environment. Journal of Visual Impairment and Blindness, 84(2): 247-249.

Brookbank, J.W. (1990). The biology of aging. Philadelphia: Harper & Row.

Carnevali, D.L. & Patrick, M. (Eds.)(1993). Nursing management for the elderly (3rd ed.). Philadelphia: J.B. Lippincott.

Carter, D.M. & Balin, A.K. (March 1983). Dermatological Aspects of Aging. Medical Clinics of North America, 67(Issue 2): 531-543.

Chinn, A.B. (Ed.).(1971). Working with older people: A guide to clinical practice (Volume IV, Clinical aspects of aging. U.S. Department of Health, Education & Welfare (Publication No. PHS-1459). U.S. Government Printing Office, Washington, DC.

Christian, E., Dluhy, N. & O'Neill, R. (1989). Sounds of silence: Coping with Hearing Loss and Loneliness. Journal of Gerontological Nursing, 15(11): 4-9.

Christian, E., Dluhy, N. & Simon, E.P. (February 1986). Visual Handicaps in the Aged: Self Reported Visual Disability and the Quality of Life of Residents of Public Housing for the Elderly. Journal of Visual Impairment and Blindness, 80(2): 588-590.

Hampton, J.K. (1991). The biology of human aging. Dubuque, I.A.: Wm. C. Brown.

Matteson, M.A. & McConnell, E.S. (1988). Gerontological nursing: Concepts and practice. Philadelphia: W.B. Saunders.

Salvage, A.V. (1991). Old people in hot water. Age/Ageing, 20(4): 233-235.

Saxon, S.V. & Etten, M.J. (1987). Physical change and aging: A guide for the helping professions (2nd Ed.) New York: Tiresias Press.

Shenefelt, P.D., & Fesnke, N.A. (1990). Aging and skin: Recognizing and managing common disorders. Geriatrics, 45(10): 57-66.

Sullivan, N. (April 1983). Vision in the Elderly. Journal of Gerontological Nursing, 8: 228-235.

United States Department of Health & Human Resources (February 1993). Management of cataracts in adults. Agency for Health Care Policy & Research (Pub. No. 93-0543), Rockville, MD.

Wolanin, M.O. & Phillips, L.R.F. (1981). Confusion: Prevention and care. St. Louis: C.V. Mosby.

Interviewing

Levinson, D.(1987). A guide to the clinical interview. Philadelphia: W.B. Saunders.

Garrett, A.(1942). Interviewing: Its principles and methods. New York: Family Service Association of America.

Burnside, I.M. (1978). Working with the elderly: group processes and techniques. North Scituate:Duxbury Press.

Butler, R.N. & Lewis, M.I. (1982). Aging and mental health. St. Louis: C.V. Mosby.

Care Planning

Carpenito, J. (1987). Nursing diagnosis: Application to clinical practice (2nd Ed). Philadelphia: J.B. Lippincott.

Carpenito, J. (1991). Nursing care plans and documentation. Philadelphia: J.B. Lippincott.

Carpenito, J. (1989). Handbook of nursing diagnosis. Philadelphia: J.B. Lippincott.-

Musculoskeletal

MODULE 3 - *THE MUSCULOSKELETAL SYSTEM*

Objectives

On completion of this module, the student should be able to:

1. describe normal age-related changes which occur in muscles, bones and supporting structures;
2. recognize the most common musculoskeletal problems and diseases of older persons;
3. detail strategies for safety and health promotion in regard to changes in the musculoskeletal system; and
4. identify symptoms of osteoarthritis, and develop a plan of care (with goals and interventions) and ways of evaluating the effectiveness of the plan.

Normal age-related changes in the musculoskeletal system

As one ages, there is a decrease in both the size and number of muscle fibres. Muscle size (also known as muscle mass) declines consistently after 30 years of age, and the decline is more rapid after age 50. Muscle flexibility and elasticity also decline. The changes are more apparent in the lower half of the body, and smooth muscle is less affected than skeletal muscle. Long term use of certain medications (such as diuretics or steroids) can deplete skeletal muscle electrolytes and contribute to muscle weakness. Inadequate (1) protein, calories, vitamin D, calcium, magnesium, zinc, B_{12}, B_6 and vitamin A; and (2) use of the muscles including too little physical activity and exercise, or being bedfast or wheelchair bound, further weaken muscles.

Bone attains its maximum density when one is between 18 and 30 years of age. After that time, bones begin to lose mass and become more porous (that is less dense). The loss occurs more rapidly in women than in men.

Extreme thinning and brittleness of the bone (a decrease in the absolute mass of bone) is known as **osteoporosis**. Decreased oestrogen levels, smoking, alcohol, lack of exercise, calcium deficiency, early menopause, possible changes in protein metabolism, and, frequent use of steroids contribute to osteoporosis. Whether osteoporosis is considered to be a typical age-related change *or* an illness probably depends on the degree of the osteoporosis.

Changes in bone also affect the spinal column. Loss of bone density in the vertebral discs causes elderly people to lose height and to have a tendency towards stooped posture. A spinal curvature known as **kyphosis** can occur.

IMPLICATIONS AND RECOMMENDATIONS

Muscle weakness in the elderly is widespread and associated with frailty, functional decline, falls, and injuries. Inactivity and undernutrition are at least partially reversible with appropriate interventions.

In countries where "sitting square" is common, problems with movement, especially in the hips, can increase dramatically with age. Regular stretching and extension of the legs is to be encouraged.

Exercise plans to improve muscle strength should be individualized and based on evaluation by a physician and physical therapist when available. The principle of strengthening involves using progressive resistance exercise (PRE) which is a gradual increase in the resistance applied to the muscle and a *small number of repetitions* to increase muscle strength. *This is a different approach from aerobic training*, which places little resistance on muscles while carrying out a large number of repetitions. Aerobic exercises tend to improve endurance rather than muscle strength, and can cause fatigue in older persons (Fiatarone & Evans, 1993; Pyka et al., 1994; Delorme, 1945).

Changes in posture and gait result from changes in the long bones and spinal column, and make older people less stable and balanced when walking. Changes in the senses such as those which occur in the eye and proprioceptors, add to the danger of falls and the likelihood of fractures.

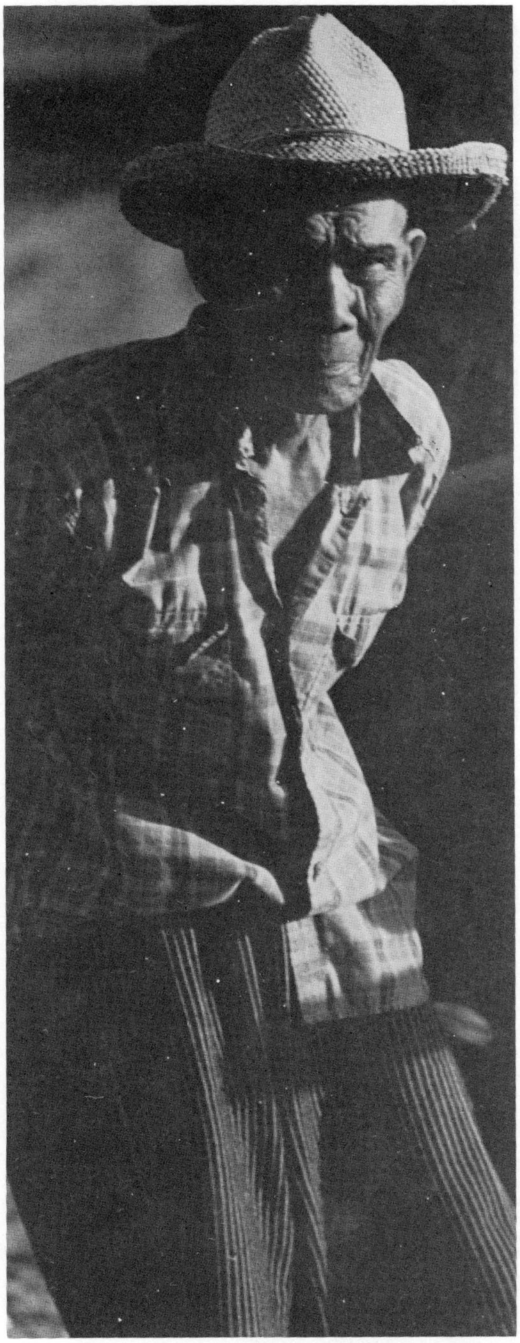

Photo courtesy of Coalition of Services for the Elderly, Inc. (COSE)

Changes in posture and gait result from changes in the long bones and spinal column. These add danger of fractures caused by falls. To create a safe environment is important.

In addition to fractures due to falls, spontaneous vertebral fractures may also occur and these cause much chronic pain for many older people.

The need to create a safe environment cannot be overemphasized.

Falls can impair the ability of older persons to care for themselves, remain independent, and to walk, exercise and remain active. Correction of nutritional inadequacies, avoidance of smoking and alcohol, and physical exercise all help to prevent further bone loss. Current treatment may include prescription of hormone replacement therapy.

NOTE: **Pain associated with fractures can interfere with sleep, and lead to decreased activity, socialization, isolation and depression.**

Decreased elasticity in the chest muscles and cartilage between ribs, make the volume of lung expansion and the reserve capacity *smaller.* Older people may tire quickly and get pneumonia more easily than younger persons. Their activities should be spread out and paced as much as possible to avoid fatigue. Early treatment of colds and flu, good nutrition, adequate exercise, no smoking and deep breathing exercises can help prevent pulmonary complications.

There are two more changes in muscles which are important to know in regard to older people. First, smaller muscles mean that older people *have less storage of glycogen* (fuel for body energy). This may mean that they have a slower reaction time for response to emergencies and crises. Second, especially in women who have had children, decreased muscle tone can make it very hard in their later years to *control urination*.

The most common diseases and illnesses

Osteoarthritis, also known as degenerative arthritis, is a non-inflammatory deterioration of joints which begins with thinning and loss of cartilage, and progresses to more complete loss of cartilage and the formation of bone spurs. The precise cause is not known but gender, genetic predisposition, obesity, wear and tear and joint trauma from injuries all contribute.

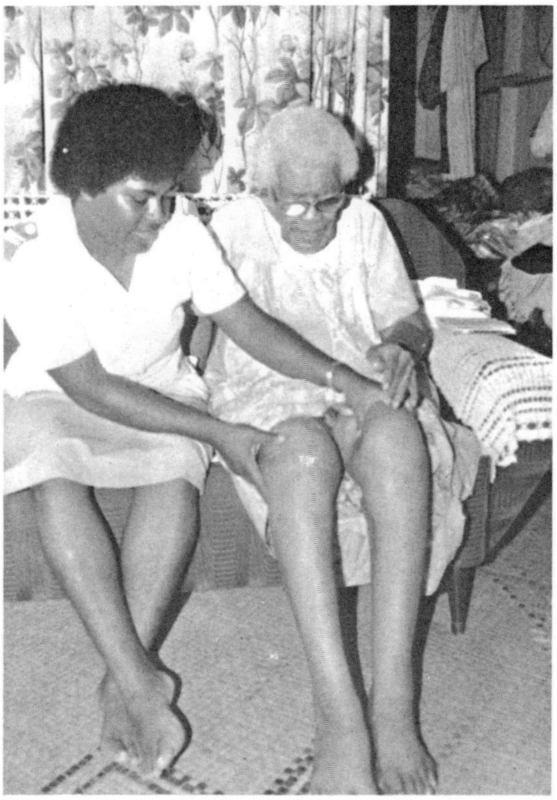

Photo courtesy of T. Miller

This Fijian lady complains of pain in her knees. She has a diagnosis of osteoarthritis. It is important that the nurse encourages her to keep mobile.

Recently, a genetic defect was identified on the number 12 gene, in family members who all had primary generalized osteoporosis. The number 12 gene is responsible for regulating Type II collagen production, the most abundant component of cartilage, the sinewy substance that stretches over the ends of bones and allows bones to glide past each other in movement without friction (Appel, 1990).

Beyond 60 years of age, about 25% of women and 15% of men have symptoms of osteoarthritis and by 75 years of age, as many as 85% may have evidence of the disease (Carnevali & Patrick, 1993).

Osteoarthritis affects mainly the weight-bearing joints (knees, hips, lower spine), cervical spine and fingers. The onset is gradual, the disease progresses slowly over years, pain is aching, morning stiffness and stiffness following inactivity such as sitting for long periods are common, nodes may appear on the hands and crepitus (creaking joints) may be heard.

Osteoarthritis should not be confused with ***rheumatoid arthritis*** which is an inflammatory process affecting persons 20 to 60 years of age and involving the lining around joints. The synovial membranes become rough, granulated and swollen, ulnar deviation of the hands is characteristic, the onset may be sudden and periods of remission are common. This disease is much more disabling and deforming than osteoarthritis and treatment usually requires use of steroids and/or other non-steroidal anti-inflammatory agents.

Hip fractures are a serious danger for older persons and can lead to major disabling illness and often lead to death. According to Brocklehurst (1976), hip fractures are typically of two types: (1) Subcapital and Transcervical Fractures, and (2) Intertrochanteric and Subtrochanteric Fractures.

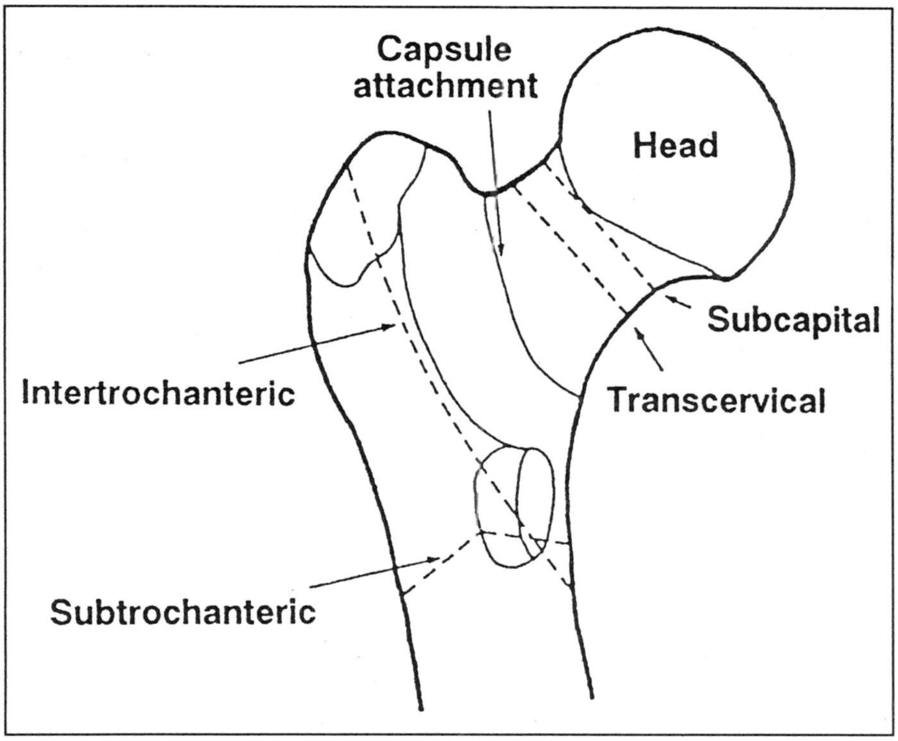

Diagramme of various types of fracture of the neck of the femur.

Subcapital and transcervical fractures

- These occur *within* the joint capsule (See illustration).
- Older persons usually do well immediately following the fracture.
- However, because the joint capsule has less blood supply than some other areas of bone, the bone takes longer to heal.

Delayed healing results in longer convalescence, extended rehabilitation and the associated risks of pneumonia, pressure sores and other problems of immobilization.

Intertrochanteric and subtrochanteric fractures

- These occur outside the joint capsule (See illustration).
- Older persons do not do as well immediately following the fracture. The explanation for this is not known, but persons with this type of fracture tend to be advanced in age.
- Because this part of the bone has greater blood supply, the healing of the bone is usually good.
- If the older person makes it successfully past the acute phase, the recovery and convalescence are shorter and better.

IMPLICATIONS AND RECOMMENDATIONS

Since there is no remission in the course of ***osteoarthritis***, interventions are aimed at alleviating symptoms (with mild analgesics) and adapting the environment so that limitations in activities of daily living (ADL) are affected as little as possible. For this reason, *it is very important that one anticipate* (that is recognize and plan ahead) what the needs will be of older persons with this condition.

Opening containers, bottles and cans will often need to be done for the older person whose hands are affected. These can be opened prior to need and then loosely placed on the top. If possible, no breakable dishes and drinking mugs should be used. Medication containers are another likely need to consider. These types of preparations help to keep the older person functioning independently for eating, taking of medications and so on.

Some forms of clothing are more easily put on than others. For example, slacks and skirts with elastic bands, and attire which slips easily over the head are more easily managed by persons with arthritis. Putting certain outfits on backwards so that they fasten in the front rather than (as intended) in the back also supports independence in dressing.

Many inexpensive assistive devices are available and/or can be easily made to modify the home environment (for example the kitchen and bathroom) and create greater independence for older people.

Periodic rest, avoidance of excessive exercise such as stair climbing, and weight loss are recommended to help relieve symptoms of osteoarthritis.

Both osteoarthritis and hip fractures can limit ability to perform activities of daily living (ADLs). They also place older people at risk for many complications.

Exercise A

Mrs. B is a 68-year old widow who has both osteoporosis and osteoarthritis, and smokes because she says it is one of the few pleasures she has left since her husband died. She is allergic to milk. She also has a heart irregularity for which she takes a cardiac medication once a day in the morning. Her memory is good but her arthritis makes it impossible for her to manage small tasks with her hands, such as opening the medicine bottle and preparing meals. She lives with her daughter who works a half day from 6:00 am until noon. Develop the plan for her including bathing, eating, taking medication, exercise, safety in the environment, quitting or limiting smoking, and exercise.

Exercise B

Role-play the following situation. Have one student take the part of an older person, refusing to bend arms and legs because of osteoarthritis. Let another student take the part of a health care worker who is trying to help the older person get dressed. Use sweaters, coats, dresses, shirts or blouses, trousers, pajamas or any other form of clothing, and attempt to get them on. Which pose the most difficulty? How can this activity of daily living be modified to make dressing easier?

Short-answer exercise

1. Changes in the musculoskeletal system affect bones, cartilage between ribs, the intervertebral discs and so on. In addition to falls, what other health and safety risks do these changes pose for older persons?

2. What are the main complications of hip fractures which occur in the intertrochanteric and subtrochanteric areas?

3. What are some ways that pain can be managed without using medication or in addition to medication? What are some of the ways in which chronic pain affects the quality of life of persons with this problem?

Students can assess and observe older people in a health care centre or community according to the list in the Assessment of practical skills section. Select older persons for the assessment and have them develop a complete plan of care.

Bibliography

Aldrich N. (Ed). (October 12, 1990). Older Americans Report, (14)40: Business Publishers Inc: Silver Spring, MD, 395.

Ali, N.S., & Bennett, S.J. (1991). Postmenoposal women. Factors in osteoporosis preventive behaviors. Journal of Gerontological Nursing, 12: 23-32.

Appel. A. (Ed)(1990). Aging news, 13(16), Silver Spring MD: Business Publishers Inc., 121.

Brocklehurst, J.C. & Hanley, T. (1976). Geriatric medicine for students. New York: Churchill Livingstone.

Brookbank, J.W. (1991). The biology of aging. Philadelphia: Harper & Row.

Carnevali, D.L. & Patrick, M. (Eds.)(1993). Nursing management for the elderly (3rd ed.) Philadelphia: J.B. Lippincott.

Chinn, A.B. (Ed.).(1971). Working with older people: A guide to clinical practice (Volume IV, Clinical aspects of aging. U.S. Department of Health, Education & Welfare (Publication No. PHS-1459). U.S. Government Printing Office, Washington, DC.

Craven, R. & Bruno P. (1986). Teach the elderly to prevent falls. Journal of Gerontological Nursing, 12(8): 27-33.

Delorme, T.L. (1945). Restoration of muscle power by heavy resitance exercises. Journal of Bone & Joint Surgury, 27(4): 645-667.

Fiatarone, M.A. & Evans, W.J. (1993). The etiology and reversibility of muscle dysfunction in the aged. The Journals of Gerontology, 48 (Special Issue): 77-83.

Holm, K. & Walker, J. (1990). Osteoporosis: Treatment and prevention update. Geriatric Nursing, 11(3): 140-142.

Kaplun, A. (Ed.)(1992). Health promotion and chronic illness: Discovering a new quality of health. Geneva: World Health organization, European Series No. 44.

Kart, C.S., Metress, E.I. & Metress, J.F. (1978). Aging & health: Biological and social perspectives. Menlo Park, CA: Addison-Wesley.

Lufkin, E.G. (1991). Paper presented at the Tenth Annual National Conference of Gerontological Nurse Practitioners, September 12, Rochester, Minn., in cooperation with the Mayo Center for Nursing.

Lufkin, E.G. & Ory, S.J. (1989). Estrogen replacement therapy for the prevention of osteoporosis. AFP, 40(3): 205-212.

Madson, S. (1989). How to reduce the risk of postmenopausal osteoporosis. Journal of Gerontological Nursing, 15(9): 20-24.

Matteson, M.A. & McConnell, E.S. (1988). Gerontological nursing: Concepts and practice. Philadelphia: W.B. Saunders.

McMahon, M.A. (1992). Osteoporosis: Identifying high-risk persons. Journal of Gerontological Nursing, 18(10): 19-26.

Pyka, G., Lindenberger, E., Charette, S. & Marcus, R. (1994). Muscle strength and fiber adaptations to a year-long resistance training program in elderly men and women. Journal of Gerontolgy, 49(1): M22-M27.

Sardana, R. (1992). Nutritional management of osteoporosis. Geriatric Nursing, 13(6): 315-319.

Saxon, S.V. & Etten, M.J. (1987). Physical change and aging: A guide for the helping professions (2nd Ed.)

Urinary

MODULE 4 - *THE URINARY SYSTEM*

Objectives

On completion of this module, the student should be able to:

1. describe normal age-related changes which occur in the urinary system;
2. screen the urinary system for normal age-related function:
   - assess the system
   - identify and prioritize alterations
   - develop care plans including goals and interventions for health promotion strategies;
3. identify common health problems, (that is deviations from expected age-related changes) in the urinary system; and
4. develop plans (with goals and interventions) for common problems, and ways of evaluating effectiveness.

Normal age-related changes in the urinary system

The number of glomeruli per kidney decreases by 30-50% between ages 25 and 85. Not only does the number of filtering units decrease but the remaining glomeruli function less well. Changes in elastin lead to calcification and thickening of arterial walls in the kidney. As a result of these changes, the **glomerular filtration rate (GFR)** *declines* nearly 50% between 20 and 90 years of age. For example, at 40 years of age the glomerular filtration rate is about 120 ml per minute and by age 85 it is only about 60 ml per minute.

The kidney becomes less responsive to sodium loss. The antidiuretic hormone (ADH), which is produced by the hypothalamus, acts to alter the permeability of certain kidney cells so that water is conserved. In older persons, there is *less effective ADH* action, less sodium is retained and therefore more water is lost.

Further, most glomerular filtration occurs in the daytime. Therefore, the greatest volume of urine is typically excreted while one is awake. In older people, this pattern is less prominent and may even be reversed. Their **kidneys** continue to be *quite active during the night*.

The bladder capacity, that is how much urine can be held before needing to urinate, decreases from 500-600 ml to about 250 ml . Not only is the capacity lower but there is more *residual* urine remaining after voiding. The smaller capacity of the bladder combined with greater night-time glomerular filtration results in the older person getting up several times during the night to urinate.

Older persons usually have less muscle tone in the abdomen (and/or in the pelvic floor due to childbirths), and these also make bladder control more difficult.

In men, enlargement of the prostate can block the flow of urine through the urethra, causing hesitancy and difficulty initiating the stream. *The problem for men* most often involves *retention of urine* or retention with overflow. *For older women*, there is generally *more difficulty* with *uncontrolled* bladder *emptying* and *leakage* of urine.

IMPLICATIONS AND RECOMMENDATIONS

There are several concerns in regard to urinary function:

- Inadequate emptying of the bladder leads to stasis (accumulation) of urine and a greater chance for urinary tract infections and the formation of stones.

- The lessened ability of ADH to adequately prevent excessive loss of fluid means that diarrhoea and vomiting conditions are likely to quickly cause serious dehydration in older persons, often with electrolyte imbalance and cardiac irregularities as well. Diuretics can have a very similar effect. Loss of sodium (which is called hyponatremia) is a frequent cause of confusion in older people.
- Many medications are excreted in the urine. Because the kidneys filter about 50% less than in younger years, drugs are not cleared as quickly in older persons. Many medications can be toxic or have excessive effects because they are being cleared slowly.
- Problems with urine control cause embarrassment and can reduce socialization.
- Incontinence causes a lot more laundry to be done, expense in supplies, unpleasant odours, potential skin irritation, and overall a difficult situation to care for in the home.
- Urgency and trying to get to the toilet in a hurry increase the chance that the older person will fall.
- Getting up frequently during the night to empty the bladder (called nocturia), interferes with sleep and needed rest, and predisposes to falls in the dark.

The most common problem of the urinary system for older people is urinary incontinence.

Urinary incontinence

Urinary incontinence can be classified as either **acute** or **chronic**. **Acute or sudden** incontinence is usually due to urinary tract infections, vaginal infections, fecal impactions, or medication use. Acute incontinence resolves as soon as the underlying cause is treated.

According to the most recent clinical protocols (USDHHS, 1992), **chronic** urinary incontinence can be classified as (1) **stress**, (2) **urge**, or (3) **overflow** according to the following definitions :

Stress incontinence is involuntary loss of urine during coughing, sneezing, laughing, or other physical activity. The symptom may be confirmed by observing urine loss during activities that incur increased abdominal pressure.

Urge incontinence is involuntary loss of urine associated with an abrupt and strong desire to void (urgency). There is usually urinary frequency, urgency, or a complaint of "I'm unable to make it to the toilet on time". At times urine loss is massive and sudden, occurring with little or no warning at all.

Overflow incontinence is involuntary loss of urine associated with overdistension of the bladder (overflow). This type of urinary incontinence may have different symptoms including frequent or constant dribbling of urine, or may include both stress or urge incontinence symptoms.

Managing incontinence

The following approaches are from Heckheimer (1989): Health Promotion of the Elderly in the Community. The interventions for managing incontinence depend on the type of incontinence problem. Although medications and surgery are sometimes needed, most symptoms can be minimized by behavioural techniques and adaptation of the environment. See the table which follows this page.

Stress incontinence does not occur at night unless the person has a lot of sneezing or coughing, or unless they have sexual activity. The first intervention is to teach Kegel exercises to the older person, to help improve the tone of the pelvic musculature.

MANAGEMENT OF URINARY INCONTINENCE

Type of incontinence	Characteristics or symptoms	Interventions/approaches	Goals
Stress	Urine leaks when one laughs, sneezes, coughs, or does physical activity Doesn't usually occur at night	• Kegel exercises* • Toilet every 2 hours • Drink 6-8 glasses of fluid per day • No fluids after 8:00 pm • Wear loose clothing	Avoid wetting accidents
Urge	Complaint of: "I'm unable to make it to the toilet on time" Loss of control of urine with little or no warning	• Anticholineric medications if ordered • Kegel exercises* • Toilet every 2 hours • Drink 6-8 glasses of fluid per day • No fluids after 8:00 pm • Use protective pads for accidents • Avoid strenuous exercise • Limit caffeine, carbonated drinks, acidic drinks and highly spiced foods • Relaxation techniques • Loose clothing for easy changing	Achieve predictable controlled urination Prevent skin breakdown Prevent odours Avoid embarassment
Overflow	Frequent or constant dribbling of urine May be post stroke or have benign prostatic hypertrophy	• Crede manoeuvre** • Drink 6-8 glasses of fluid per day • No fluids after 8:00 pm • Monitor for UTI • Change damp clothes frequently • Catheterize if ordered	Prevent urinary tract infections
Functional	Mental confusion Lack of urine control - in regard to timing and location	• Regular toileting every 2 to 3 hours • Frequently change wet clothes • Skin care • Hygiene measures	

* See page 6.
**See page 7.

To do **Kegel** exercises do the following:

Have the older person begin and stop the stream of urine every time s/he empties the bladder. This should be done several times during each visit to the toilet.

S/he should also be instructed to lie or sit down, tighten the anal sphincter, hold it for about 5 seconds, release and repeat the exercise several times throughout the day. To explain how it is done, it is helpful to describe the anal sphincter control as squeezing the buttocks as if trying to prevent a bowel movement.

Additionally, the older person should:

- train the bladder by going to the toilet regularly, perhaps as often as every 2 to 3 hours, even if the urge is not felt;
- drink at least 6 to 8 glasses of fluid during the day and early evening, stopping further drinking by about 8:00 in the evening; and
- wear loose clothing so getting clothes off quickly is not a problem.

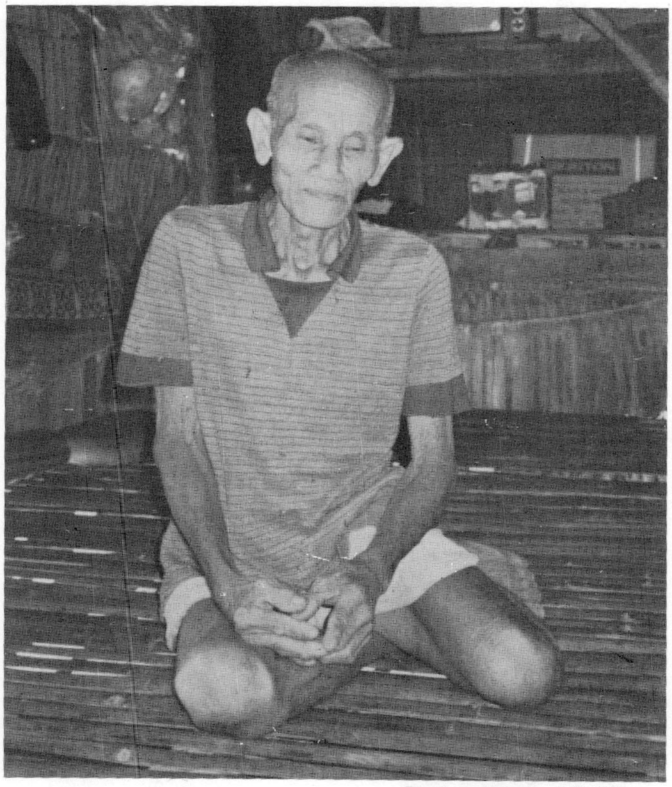

Photo courtesy of Dr Bilous

This 80-year old man in Cambodia rests on a bamboo mat in the family home. The bamboo mat provides an environment that is easily cleaned. Health workers that visit the home of the elderly should assess the urinary pattern of the older person and advise the family of the importance of good personal hygiene and methods to handle frequency of urination or incontinence.

With **urge incontinence**, older people feel the urge to urinate but have trouble getting to the toilet quickly enough. Bladder spasms contribute; therefore, anticholinergic medications are often prescribed.

NOTE: *Anticholinergic drugs* cannot be given to people with **wide angle** *glaucoma*.

In addition to medications prescribed, performing the Kegel exercises, drinking adequate fluid, and limiting fluids in the evening*, urge incontinence should be managed* by having the older person:

- avoid delay in getting to the toilet and emptying the bladder; this is done best by going to the toilet every 2 hours even if the urge is not felt;
- use some form of protection because leakage and accidents are common;
- wear loose clothing so changing clothes is easier;
- avoid strenuous exercise; and
- limit the use of dietary irritants such as caffeine, carbonated drinks, highly acidic and highly spiced foods.

NOTE: **Sometimes relaxation techniques are helpful and can be taught to *older people who have incontinence.***

With **overflow incontinence** there is constant dripping of small amounts of urine because the bladder is usually full. Because the bladder stays full and the kidneys filter during the night, there is a large volume of urine in the morning. Emptying of the bladder is generally incomplete so urinary infection is a danger with this type of incontinence. Neurogenic bladder and benign prostatic hypertrophy are causes of overflow.

Surgery or drugs may be indicated. *Other interventions for overflow incontinence include*:

- use of the **Crede** manoeuvre.

To do the **Crede** manoeuvre, have the person tighten the abdominal muscles and apply gentle downward pressure from the top of the bladder down toward the toes and repeat several times.

- drink adequate fluid and limit fluids in the evening;
- monitor for symptoms of urinary tract infection (UTI);
- change damp clothes frequently; and
- catheterization is sometimes necessary.

One additional type of incontinence is frequent and this type is called **functional incontinence**. Older persons who are incontinent as a result of confusion would be in this category. All the preceding interventions depend on the cooperation of the affected person. This partnership is not possible with someone who is cognitively impaired. Therefore, interventions are aimed at (1) regular toileting every 2 to 3 hours to catch at least some of the incontinence even if this happens by chance, (2) frequent changing of wet clothing, (3) good skin care, and (4) good hygiene.

> **REMEMBER:** *Urine is acidic and persons with incontinence are frequently wet. Good skin care is important to prevent breakdown and attention to hygiene is important to avoid odours and embarrassment.*

Exercise A

Mrs. K is 72 years old and has 7 children. She is a very active woman who participates in many activities outside of the home. She drinks a lot of coffee (or tea as the case applies) and this keeps her energy high. She and her husband have a comfortable life. However, she is having trouble with leakage of urine. She believes this is a normal part of aging, so all she does is wear a protective pad and worry about odour. Sometimes urine leaks out when she is sexually active with her husband. Develop a thorough plan of care to help her.

Exercise B

Role-play the following situation. Have one student take the part of an older woman whose urinary incontinence is causing problems with sexual activity. Have another student take the part of the husband. Have a third student take the part of the health care worker. Explore the emotional reactions of the older couple to the stated problem, and identify strategies to help them regain a satisfactory way of managing their sexual activity.

Short-answer exercise

1. Changes in kidney function affect metabolism and excretion of medications. Briefly describe how.

2. Describe how and what activities of daily living (ADLs) can be affected by urinary incontinence in women.

Suggested field experience for assessment of practical skills

Students can go to a health care centre or community to observe and assess older persons for urinary problems. Find interesting ones (perhaps women would be most suitable) and have them develop the plan of care following the on-site experience.

Bibliography

Carnevali, D.L. & Patrick, M. (Eds.)(1993). Nursing management for the elderly (3rd ed.). Philadelphia: J.B. Lippincott.

Hampton, J.K. (1991). The biology of human aging. Dubuque, IA: Wm. C. Brown.

Heckheimer, E.F. (1989). Health promotion of the elderly in the community. Philadelphia: W.B. Saunders.

Kane, R.L., Ouslander, J.G. & Abrass, I.B.(1984). Essentials of clinical geriatrics. New York: McGraw-Hill.

Kee, C.C. (1992). Age-related changes in the renal system. Causes, consequences and nursing implications. Geriatric Nursing, 13(2): 80-83, 89, 93.

Matteson, M.A. & McConnell, E.S. (1988). Gerontological nursing: Concepts and practice. Philadelphia: W.B. Saunders.

Saxon, S.V. & Etten, M.J. (1987). Physical change and aging: A guide for the helping professions (2nd Ed.) New York: Tiresias Press.

Staab, A. & Lyles, M. (1990). Manual of geriatric nursing. Glenview, IL: Scott, Foresman & Company.

Unites States Department of Health & Human Services (1992). Urinary incontinence in adults. Agency for Health Care Policy & Research, PHS (Publication No. AHCPR 92-0041, Rockville, MD: author.

Gastrointestinal

MODULE 5 - *THE GASTROINTESTINAL SYSTEM*

Objectives

On completion of this module, the student should be able to:

1. describe normal age-related changes which occur in the gastrointestinal (GI) system;
2. screen the GI system for normal age-related function:
    - assess the system
    - identify and assign priority to any dysfunction
    - develop care plans including goals and interventions for health promotion strategies;
3. identify common health problems, (that is deviations from expected age-related changes) in the GI system; and
4. develop plans (with goals and interventions) for common problems, and ways of evaluating effectiveness.

Normal age-related changes in the gastrointestinal system

In the **mouth**, the oral mucosa atrophies and the underlying connective tissue degenerates with age, causing the gums to recede around the base of the teeth. Tooth enamel becomes harder and teeth appear more translucent. Reabsorption of bone in the jaws may lead to loosening of teeth. There is decreased secretion of saliva and it becomes thicker.

Peristaltic action in the **oesophagus** is less effective, thus there is delayed entry of food into the stomach. There is decreased hydrochloric acid in the stomach. Between 40 and 60 years of age, gastric secretions may drop substantially.

The **liver** decreases in weight and function and is less able to metabolize drugs and hormones. The **large intestine** itself experiences no major change, but there is decreased tone and loss of elasticity in abdominal muscles which support peristalsis in the large bowel.

IMPLICATIONS AND RECOMMENDATIONS

In combination with changes in taste and smell perception, changes in the mouth and gums can lessen the *appetite* (that is the desire for food) of older persons. Discomfort from exposed dentin on teeth or poorly fitting dentures can make chewing painful. This generally results in either *reduced food intake* or modification of the diet to *soft foods.* In either case, nutritional status can be negatively affected. Additionally, less hydrochloric acid in the stomach can hamper the *absorption* of iron, calcium and B_{12}. Dietary instruction should be given to the family and the older person regarding ways in which food can be easily chewed and digested while still remaining nutritious. For example, cooked cereals are

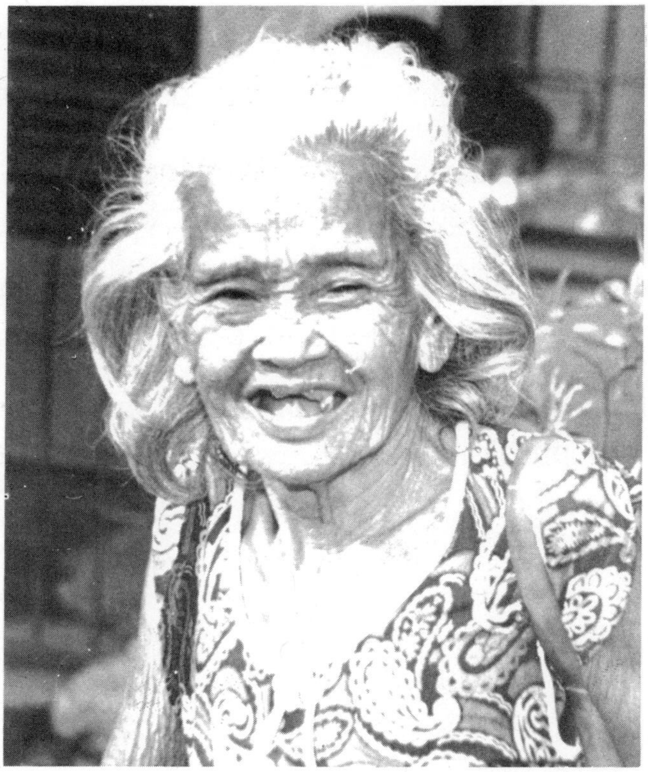

Photo courtesy of T. Miller

Changes in the mouth and gums can lessen the appetite and digestion. Dietary information should be given to the family and the elderly person regarding ways to prepare food that can be easily chewed and digested while still remaining nutritious.

a good source of fibre and are also easy to chew. Dentures should be refitted periodically.

Decreased peristalsis in the oesophagus makes older people choke more easily. Foods should be eaten in small amounts, slowly and with adequate fluid to aid swallowing.

Less hydrochloric acid in the stomach also causes reduced solubility of acidic drugs such as aspirin. Decreased liver metabolism means that medications stay longer in the body. Monitoring of medications and adjustment of doses is very important. *Families and the older members of families should be taught the possible side effects of all drugs taken.* Due to changes in the liver, tolerance for alcohol is decreased, and should therefore be avoided except in very small amounts.

Frequent health problems of the GI system in older persons

Hiatus hernia is a protrusion of the stomach into the thoracic cage through an opening in the diaphragm. It increases after age 50 and may be present in as many as 67% of persons over age 60. It is more common in women. Symptoms include heart burn, dysphagia (difficulty in swallowing), pain in the region of lower sternum, belching, reflux of food and vomiting. Interventions to correct the situation include:

- weight loss if the person is obese;
- a diet of small, frequent feedings of bland but nutritious food; avoid chocolate, coffee, tea and colas, and reduce the amount of saturated fat;
- walking for a while after eating rather than lying down, and avoiding eating prior to going to bed;
- sleeping in a semi-upright position using 2-3 pillows; and
- taking antacids for relief of heartburn; skim milk can also help.

Cancer of the **colon** and rectum increase with age. Cancer of the **colon** *is more common in women* and cancer of the *rectum is more common in men.* Symptoms include change in bowel habits (new onset constipation or diarrhoea, decreased size of stool or blood in stool), loss of appetite (anorexia), wasting, weight loss, weakness, and dull pain radiating to the back which can be relieved by bending. The mortality associated with this disease is high. Colon/rectal exams are recommended for screening for cancer. Digital rectal exam and examination of stool to check for occult (hidden) blood should be a part of routine health checks for people over 40 years of age. For people over 50 years of age, a proctoscopic examination should be considered every three to five years.

The incidence of cancer of the mouth, stomach and liver also increase with age. For some nationalities, the occurrence of these is higher than others, probably due to dietary factors. Oral screening for sores and other signs of cancer should be done, especially among persons who are at high risk from smoking, chewing tobacco, and drinking alcohol or especially hot beverages regularly.

Older persons frequently complain of **constipation** and often actually have more constipation than younger persons. However, this problem is *not* a function of normal aging since there are few age-related changes in the gastrointestinal (GI) tract. Bowel motility does not decrease with age. Instead, the difficulty with bowel actions in the elderly is thought to be related to (1) poor dietary habits including not eating enough roughage, not drinking enough fluid and having difficulty chewing, (2) too little physical activity and exercise, (3) being effected by chronic diseases that impair neural control, (4) laxative abuse and the side effects of medications, (5) limitations in functional ability, and (6) environmental barriers. Psychological factors such as depression and dementia, and myths about constipation in older persons can all predispose the elderly to constipation.

Most older people *eat less,* in part because their metabolic requirements are less; muscle mass and basal metabolic rate decline with age. It is uncertain whether taste and smell decline enough with age to interfere with the enjoyment of eating. It takes more flavor or spice to stimulate taste, but there are more than enough tastebuds to provide stimulation. The *perception* of how things taste may be impaired by age-related changes in smell. Many older persons have *difficulty with chewing*, thereby limiting their nutritional intake and causing them to avoid needed high fibre foods. Many don't eat even the minimum recommended daily servings of fruits and vegetables. Diets high in fibre help prevent constipation, and decrease the need for laxatives.

Poor fluid intake also contributes to constipation. Older people frequently drink too little, especially if they are frail, bedridden or confused. Older persons sometimes reduce their fluid intake because they fear they will be incontinent of urine.

Those who *don't take regular exercise* have more problems with constipation. Elderly people who are up and about have been found to have normal transit times (that is the time it takes for food to progress through the gut) while bedridden patients have delayed movement of bowel products (Brocklehurst, 1980). Chronic disease can lead to limitations in ambulation and activity, thereby reducing use of abdominal muscles necessary to expel stool products.

Many kinds of *medications* make bowel action difficult including diuretics, anticholinergics, opiates, and antidepressants, and the elderly typically take one or more of these. The more chronic the disease, the greater the chance that the person uses more than one medication, and the greater the likelihood of constipation. Older adults often take laxatives on a regular basis and when this happens, the body becomes dependent upon their use.

Functional disability increases with age. Therefore, older persons often need help getting on and off the toilet and in cleaning themselves after bowel actions. *Lack of privacy* and the *need for help from others* is embarrassing and may cause older persons to try to ignore the urge to defecate. If they do this repeatedly, the rectum loses its sensitivity to the urge to defecate, resulting in constipation.

There is some evidence that persons who are *depressed* have more problems with constipation, possibly because their sad state makes them less physically active. It is also possible that feeling depressed may make their appetitie poor, thus lowering their intake of food and fluids. Dementia is frequently associated with constipation in older people, probably because they are unable to communicate their need for toileting when the need arises.

Myths about constipation and older people are common. Constipation is often considered to be inevitable, resulting in older persons using laxatives routinely, and causing health care workers not to pay attention to the problem.

Constipation is not a part of normal age-related changes.

Normal bowel movements are characterized by regular, easy, and complete passage of formed stool approximately three times per week, although longer periods in between may be normal for some persons.

Symptoms of constipation include infrequent and/or incomplete evacuation, small amount of stool, difficulty pushing the stool out because it is very hard, rectal pain, severe flatus/gas, and abdominal bloating or fullness.

IMPLICATIONS AND RECOMMENDATIONS

A large number of constipated older persons develop *faecal impaction*, and this can lead to confusional states, urinary tract infection and/or incontinence, and enlargement of the lower colon. If this occurs, the hardened stool must be removed manually. This is unpleasant, embarrassing and can cause rectal bleeding.

All efforts should be focused on *prevention* of constipation. This is done by (1) assessing for risk factors and then (2) correcting the underlying cause.

The Elimination Assessment Instrument (EAI)(Sheehy, 1994) is a screening instrument in early stages of testing, but one which may help to identify and predict older persons who may be at risk for developing constipation (p. 8). Lower scores indicate more normal stools (that is the absence of factors associated with constipation) and higher scores should alert one to a tendency towards constipation.

Although the screen gives a *warning of risk* for constipation, *it does not give the cause*. Therefore, if a high score is obtained, further assessment as to contributing causes is warranted in order to individualize a plan of care. For example, look at questions number 5, 6 and 7 on the EAI. If the older person does not eat a well-balanced diet especially in terms of fibre, it is necessary to evaluate what is causing this problem, such as: lack of appetite, trouble swallowing, inadequate money to purchase food and so on.

Instructors please note that the full Nutrition screening manual is available to you at the back of this training manual.

Exercise A

Mr. T has worked hard all his life and now is happy to just sit and watch television all day. His wife died a few years ago, and since then he has been shopping for and preparing most of his own meals. He seems to be sad quite a lot too. There is little roughage in his meals because he finds some foods hard to chew. He has a little trouble with leakage of urine, so he now limits his fluid a lot. He is functioning well except for an increasing problem with constipation. Develop a thorough plan of care to help him.

Exercise B

Role-play the following situation. An older person is having problems with constipation, and the thing of most concern to him/her is that he/she has a lot of flatus (gas). Have one student play the part of the older person and another take the part of the health care worker. As a group, analyse (1) how well the health care worker responded to the feelings of embarrassment of the older person, (2) how thorough the assessment was, and (3) whether the suggestions made to the older person were sensitive to this type of concern.

Short-answer exercise

1. Changes in the peristaltic action of the oesophagus creates a choking danger for older people. Which foods commonly eaten in your country would pose the greatest danger? What foods can be substituted? What further measures should be taken?

2. It is well known that lack of exercise contributes to problems of constipation. How could one increase the exercise of an older person who is in a wheelchair?

Suggested field experience for assessment of practical skills

Students can go to a health care centre or community to observe and assess older persons for the problem of constipation. The Elimination assessment instrument following this page can be used in addition to other questions asked which are contained in the Assessment of Practical Skills in the Student evaluation tools section of the manual. Have students develop a complete plan of care together with the elderly person him/herself and the family.

Elimination Assessment Instrument

Name________________ Date of Examination________________

Does the older person:

1. Walk frequently during the day?
   (Score yes even if walking is done with physical assistance, or aids such as walkers, or canes)
   ☐ yes = 0 ☐ no = 1

2. Accomplish bowel movements independently such as getting on and off a bedpan, commode or toilet, getting or using toilet paper or hand washing?
   ☐ yes = 0 ☐ no = 1

3. Describe bowel movements as being:
   ☐ normal = 0 **OR** ☐ constipated = 1

4. Have bowel movements:
   ☐ daily or every other day= 0 ☐ every 3rd day or less frequently = 1

5. Eat a diet which is?
   ☐ regular = 0 **OR** ☐ soft = 1

6. Eat at least one serving of fresh fruit or cooked vegetables daily?
   ☐ yes = 0 ☐ no = 1

7. Eat high fibre foods such as brown rice, taro, wheat bran etc., at least twice per week?
   ☐ yes = 0 ☐ no = 1

8. Eat without supervision or is there a need for someone to feed?
   (Score yes even if food must be set up or eaten with adaptive utensils)
   ☐ yes = 0 ☐ no = 1

9. Drink at least eight (8) glasses of fluid daily?
   ☐ yes = 0 ☐ no = 1

10. Have a good appetite?
    ☐ yes = 0 ☐ no = 1

__________ ***TOTAL SCORE***

Sheehy, C.M. (1994). Development of an instrument to measure alterations in patterns of elimination among elders. Journal of Nursing Measurement. (Under Review).

Bibliography

Alessi, C.A., & Henderson, C.T. (1988). Constipation and fecal impaction in the long-term care patient. Clinics in Geriatric Medicine, 4(3): 571-588.

Anderson, J. (1984). Bowel function in the elderly. Nursing Times, 80(33): 52.

Battle, E.H., & Hanna, C.E. (1980). Evaluation of a dietary regimen for chronic constipation: Report of a pilot study. Journal of Gerontological Nursing, 6(9): 527-532.

Beverly, L., & Travis, L. (1992). Constipation: Proposed natural laxative mixture. Journal of Gerontological Nursing, 18(10): 5-12.

Bradford, L. (1988). Elimination: Bowels. In I.M. Burnside (Ed.), Nursing and the Aged (3rd ed.), (pp. 521-538). New York: McGraw Hill.

Brookbank, J.W.(1990). The biology of aging. New York: Harper & Row.

Cefalu, C.A., McKnight, G.T., & Pike, J.I. (1981). Treating impaction: A practical approach to an unpleasant problem. Geriatrics, 36(5): 143-146.

Cheskin, L.J. (1991). Constipation and diarrhea. In L.R. Barker,J.R. Burton, & P.D. Zeive (Eds.), Principles of ambulatory medicine (pp. 443-467). Baltimore: Williams & Wilkins.

Cimprich, B. (1985). Symptom management: Constipation. Cancer Nursing, 8(Suppl. 1): 39-43.

Cummings, J.H., Branch, W., Jenkins, D.J.A., Southgate, D.A.T., Houston, H., & James, W.P.T. (1978). Colonic response to dietary fibre from carrot, cabbage, apple, bran, and guar gum. Lancet, 1(8054): 5-9.

Darnton-Hill, I. (1992). Psychological aspects of nutrition and aging. Nutrition Reviews, 50(12) 476-479.

Donald, I.P., Smith, R.G., Cruikshank, J.G., Elton, R.A., & Stoddart, M.E. (1985). A study of constipation in the elderly living at home. Gerontology, 31(2): 112-118.

Ellickson, E.B. (1988). Bowel management plan for the homebound elderly. Journal of Gerontological Nursing, 14(1): 16-19.

Fedail, S.S., Badi, S.M., & Musa, A.R.M. (1984). The effects of sorghum and wheat bran on the colonic functions of healthy Sudanese subjects. The American Journal of Clinical Nutrition, 40(4): 776-779.

Fich, A., Camilleri, M., & Phillips, S.F. (1989). Effect of age on human gastric and small bowel motility. Journal of Clinical Gastroenterology, 11(4): 416-420.

Finlay, M. (1988). The use of dietary fibre in a long-stay geriatric ward. Journal of Nutrition for the Elderly, 8(1): 19-30.

Fisher, M. (Ed.)(1989). Guide to clinical preventive services: An assessment of the effectiveness of 169 interventions (Report of the US Preventive Services Task Force). Baltimore, MD: Williams & Wilkins.

Fleischer, D. E. et al. (1989). Detection and surveillance of colorectal cancer. Journal of the American Medical Association, 262(4): 580-585.

Graham, D.Y., Moser, S.E., & Estes, M.K. (1982). The effects of bran on bowel function in constipation. American Journal of Gastroenterology, 77(9): 599-603.

Groth, F. (1988). Effects of wheat bran in the diet of postsurgical orthopaedic patients to prevent constipation. Orthopaedic Nursing, 7(4): 41-46.

Hale, W.E., Perkins, L.L., May, F.E., Marks, R.G. & Stewart, R.B.(1986). Symptom prevalence in the elderly: An evaluation of age, sex, disease, and medication use. Journal of the American Geriatrics Society, 34(5): 333-340.

Hope, A. (1983). The relief of constipation in the elderly. The Australian Nurses' Journal, 12(10): 45-48.

Hull, C., Greco, R.S., & Brooks, D.L. (1980). Alleviation of constipation in the elderly by dietary fiber supplementation. Journal of the American Geriatrics Society, 28(9): 410-414.

Lieberman, D.A. (1990). Colon cancer screening. Archives of Internal Medicine, 150(April): 740-744.

Lindsey, A.M. (1983). Phenomena and physiological variables of relevance to nursing, review of a decade of work: Part II. Western Journal of Nursing Research, 5(1): 41-63.

McShane, R.E. & McLane, A.M. (1985). Constipation: Consensual and empirical validation. Nursing Clinics of North America, 20(4): 801-808.

Meza, J.P., Peggs, J.F. & O'Brien, J.M. (1984). Constipation in the elderly patient. The Journal of Family Practice, 18(5): 695-703.

Milne, J.S., & Williamson, J. (1972). Bowel habit in older people. Gerontologica Clinica, 14(1): 56-60.

Morley, J.E., Mooradian, A.D., Silver, A.J., Heber, D. & Alfin-Slater, R.B. (1988). Nutrition in the elderly. Annals of Internal Medicine, 109(11): 890-904.

Nutrition Screening Initiative (1991). Report of nutrition screening 1: Toward a common view. April 8-10, Washington, DC: Author.

Pringle, R., Pennington, M.J., Pennington, C.R., & Ritchie, R.T. (1984). A study of the influence of a fibre biscuit on bowel function in the elderly. Age & Ageing, 13(3): 175-178.

Read, N.W. & Timms, J.M. (1986). Defecation and the pathophysiology of constipation. Clinics in Gastroenterology, 15(4): 934-965.

Read, N.W., & Timms, J. M. (1987). Constipation: Is there a light at the end of the tunnel? Scandanavian Journal of Gastroenterology, 129(Supplement): 88-96.

Rose, J.D.R., Troughton, A.H., Harvey, J.S. & Smith, P.M.(1986). Depression and functional bowel disorders in gastrointestinal outpatients. Gut, 27(9): 1025-1028.

Schmelzer, M. (1990). Effectiveness of wheat bran in preventing constipation of hospitalized orthopaedic surgery patients. Orthopaedic Nursing, 9(6): 55-59.

Schuster, M.M. (1983). Colonic motor dysfunction and incontinence in the aging patient. In E.C. Texter (Ed.), The aging gut (pp. 166-172). New York: Masson Publishing.

Shamburek, R.D. & Farrar, J.T. (1990). Disorders of the digestive system in the elderly. New England Journal of Medicine, 322(7): 438-443.

Shamburek, R.D., Scott, R.B. & Farrar, J.T. (1990). Gastrointestinal and liver changes in the elderly. In Geriatric surgery: Comprehensive care of the elderly patient. (pp.97-113), Mark R. Katlic (Ed.), Baltimore, MD: Urban & Schwarzenberg.

Sheehy, C.M. (1994). Development of an instrument to measure alterations in patterns of elimination among elders. Journal of Nursing Measurement, (under review).

Shreeve, C. (1985). Bowel habits in the elderly. Nursing Mirror, 160(19): 20-21.

Sklar, J. (1983). Gastrointestinal diseases in the aged. In W. Reichel (Ed.) Clinical Aspects of Aging (pp. 205-217). Baltimore: Williams & Wilkins.

Stewart, R.B., Moore, M.T., & Marks, R.G. (1992). Correlates of constipation in an ambulatory elderly population. American Journal of Gastroenterology, 87: 859-864.

Suboticanec, K., Stavijenic, A., Bilic-Pesic, L., Gorajscan, M., Gorajscan, D., Brubacher, G. & Buzina, R. (1989). Nutritional status, grip strength, and immune function in institutionalized elderly. International Journal for Vitamin & Nutrition Research, 59(1): 20-28.

Talley, N.J., Camilleri, M., Orkin, B.A. & Kramlinger, K.G.(1989). Effect of cyclical unipolar depression on upper gastrointestina l motility and sleep. Gastroenterology, 97(3): 775-777.

Wald, A. (1986). Colonic transit and anorectal manometry in chronic idiopathic constipation. Archives of Internal Medicine, 146(9): 1713-1716.

Cardiovascular/
Respiratory

MODULE 6 - *CARDIOVASCULAR AND RESPIRATORY SYSTEMS*

Objectives

On completion of this module, the student should be able to:

1. describe normal age-related changes which occur in the cardiovascular and respiratory systems;
2. list common health problems, (that is deviations from expected age-related changes) in the cardiovascular and respiratory systems;
3. develop plans (with goals and interventions) for the management of such common health problems; and
4. develop plans (with goals and interventions) for health promotion for cardiopulmonary fitness.

Normal age-related changes

Cardiovascular system

As one gets older, the heart works harder but less efficiently. The pulse increases because of more frequent contractions, but the contractions are weaker and therefore the amount of blood pumped to the body with each beat is less.

The amount of interstitial fibrous tissue and fat surrounding the heart increases. The heart valves become thicker and less elastic. Peripheral vascular resistance increases, i.e. it is harder for the blood to pass through the blood vessels. Changes in collagen and elastin make the blood vessels more rigid and less elastic, and fatty deposits appear. These changes occur over a lifetime, and are caused or aggravated by diets high in saturated fats and low in fibre, poor exercise patterns and smoking.

Pacemaker cells appear to decline. The conduction system may be more susceptible to irritabilities, and non-life threatening extra beats may be more common.

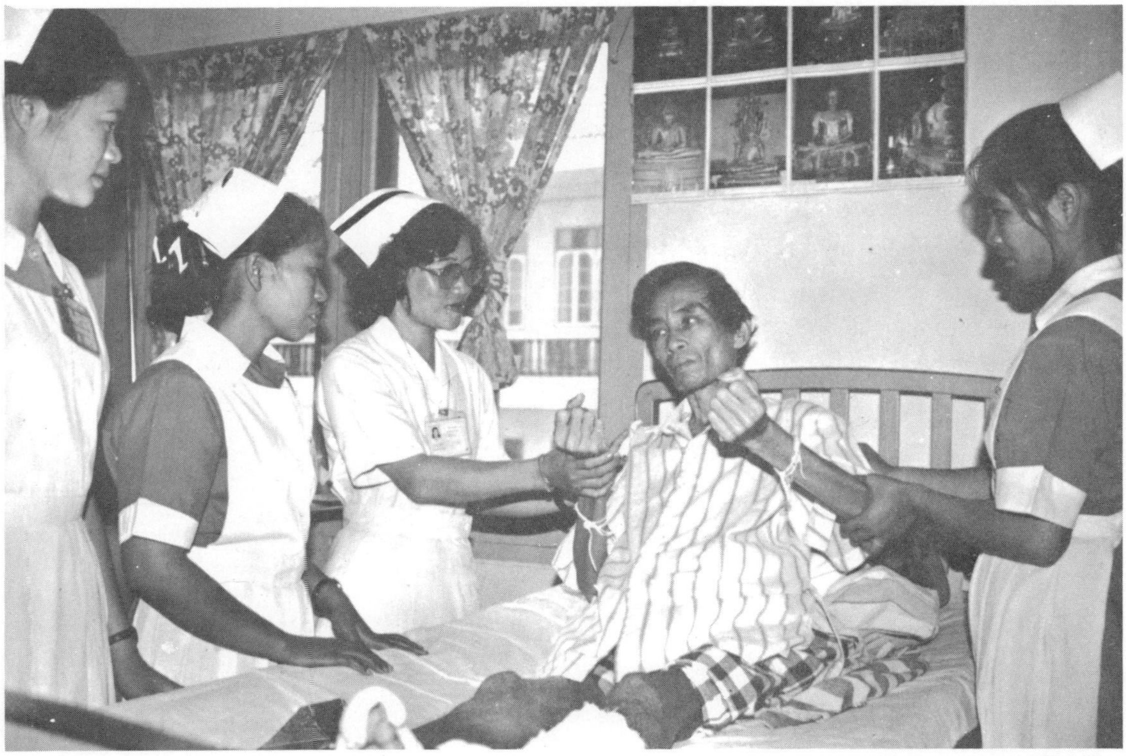

Photo courtesy of T. Miller

Student nurses and families who care for bed-ridden persons in the Lao People's Democratic Republic are taught the importance of regular physical exercise to minimise the risk of deformities, and promotion of oxygen transportation to all parts of the body.

Overall, there is little functional consequence to the changes in the cardiovascular system except under conditions of stress. When challenged (such as with heavy exercise or a rapid change in position from lying to standing), *the heart responds less effectively to the stress, and takes longer to return to normal.* Normally in younger persons, when the demand for circulation rises in response to the existence of stress, the heart beats more strongly but at a lower rate.

Respiratory system

Lung tissue becomes less elastic and there is less strength in respiratory muscles and the diaphragm. The rib cage becomes stiffer and more rigid. Alveoli increase in size and decrease in number; therefore there is less alveolar surface and less effective exchange of oxygen and carbon dioxide. The size or *depth* of the *maximum breath* which one can take *becomes smaller.*

There is also a decrease in the cough reflex and in ciliary action in the lungs.

All these changes are worsened by smoking or heavy air pollution.

IMPLICATIONS AND RECOMMENDATIONS

Changes in the cardiovascular system make older persons more susceptible to fainting (**orthostatic hypotension**) with sudden change in position, for example when moving from a lying to an upright position.

The greater tendency for fainting means there is a greater chance of falls and other injuries. Older persons should be instructed to change positions slowly, remaining seated until the body adjusts, and then coming to a fully upright position. Changes in the arteries make the risk of **stroke** (**cerebrovascular accident**) and associated loss of independence greater. Even if lifelong health habits have not been positive, beginning more healthy behaviour can reduce the risk of stroke. Quitting or at least reducing smoking and drinking of alcohol, lowering fat and salt and increasing soluble bran in the diet, and exercising regularly are all recommended.

Angina (chest pain with activity), **palpitations**, **heart blocks**, **congestive heart failure**, **heart attacks** and many other cardiac diseases become more likely.

It is becoming increasingly clear that suitable exercise is appropriate throughout life, including in the elderly, and has many benefits, including reducing morbidity from cardiovascular disease. This important issue, along with diet and not smoking, is considered again in module 12.

Medications need to be monitored carefully and the potential side effects taught to older persons and their families. Medications such as digitalis preparations and diuretics require particular care because their action is very much affected by age-related changes in the kidney, liver, muscle mass and fat and fluid distribution.

The decrease in cilia and cough action, along with changes in the immune system, reduce the effectiveness of gas exchange and make the older person more susceptible to **Pneumonia**. Distinct symptoms (such as fever, lung pain or productive cough) often do not accompany pneumonia in older adults. *The symptoms are typically vague such as fatigue or confusion.* Other respiratory problems such as **chronic obstructive lung disease**, **emphysema**, **chronic bronchitis** and **asthma** also increase with age, especially among the elderly with a history of smoking.

The amount of exercise or activity that can be tolerated is less. Activities should be spaced with rest periods. The benefit of regular moderate exercise such as walking and aerobic activity should be emphasized.

Another important respiratory problem for the elderly is **Tuberculosis**. Because the tuberculosis bacilli are extremely hardy, they often remain viable within a healthy host for years. Three symptoms bring to mind tuberculosis: weight loss, rise of temperature (modest) and chronic cough (more than three weeks).

The association of these symptoms or chronic cough alone are investigated by repeated sputum examinations (three). A positive result (bacilli present in the sputum by direct examination or by culture) confirms the diagnosis. A negative result does not deny the diagnosis. Further investigations are done. WHO policy advice is to treat chronic cough with no mycobacteria in the sputum with non-specific antibiotics for 15 days. If there is improvement (no temperature, weight gain, improvement of cough) the tuberculosis diagnosis is no longer evoked. If there is no improvement, a chest X-ray should be done to confirm the diagnosis.

BCG is preventing the occurrence of the more serious forms of the disease in children and protecting against tuberculosis in a range of 20-80% of potential cases depending on the country.

Treatment of tuberculosis is standardized and uses four drugs in the initial phase (two months) and two in the continuation phase (four or six months). This treatment, called short-course chemotherapy (SCC) is highly effective (85-99% of patients are cured) if taken properly.

Dosages in the treatment of the elderly have to be carefully adjusted and kidney function has to be checked whenever possible.

Exercise

Enact the following situation in a role play. You have been asked to develop a specific, individualized plan for cardiovascular fitness for Mrs D. She is more than a little overweight, loves to eat chocolates and cheese, and has no real hobbies except food. She does not smoke but she does live in an area where the air is very polluted. When asked why she doesn't exercise more, she says, "It will only make me breathe more of that polluted air." Her son says that she will be hard to motivate because she barely leaves her house. Develop a plan for her which is realistic. Be certain to write interventions about how you will *motivate* her.

Short-answer exercise

1. Mr. L seems to be doing fine. However, of his brothers, father and grandfather, no one has lived past 62 years of age. Mr. L is now 58 years old and has been retired for six months. His wife is concerned that he is not active enough. He claims, "I've worked hard my entire life. I deserve to rest." Respond to this scenario.

2. The family of Mrs. C tells you their mother has had a cold for several weeks and she feels fatigued. They cannot describe any specific symptoms that cause them concern, but the family is convinced that Mrs. C is acting a bit confused. This is not normal for Mrs. C, who has no history of dementing illness. She has not been prescribed (and is not taking) any medications which might cause confusion nor is she taking any medications for the cold symptoms. Describe what illness might be the cause of Mrs. C's symptoms and what to do.

Suggested field experience for assessment of practical skills

Students can be placed in a health centre or community to observe and assess a variety of cardiovascular and respiratory changes and problems. Select an older person of particular interest and have students develop a complete plan of care.

Bibliography

Brookbank, J.W.(1990). The biology of aging. New York: Harper & Row.

Carnevali, D.L. & Patrick, M. (Eds.)(1993). Nursing management for the elderly (3rd ed.). Philadelphia: J.B. Lippincott.

Close, L.G., & Wodson, G.E. (1989). Common upper airway disorders in the elderly and their management. Geriatrics, 44(1): 67-72.

Dutt, A.K. & Stead, W.W. (1992). Tuberculosis. Clinics in Geriatric Medicine, 8(4): 771-775.

Evans, J.G. & Williams, T.F. (Eds.)(1992). Oxford textbook of geriatric medicine. Oxford: Oxford University Press.

Hampton, J.K. (1991). The biology of human aging. Dubuque, IA: Wm. C. Brown.

Havlir, D.V., van der Kuyp, F., Duffy, E., Marshall, R., Hom, D. & Ellner, J.J. (1991). A 19-year follow-up of tuberculin reactors: Assessment of skin test reactivity and in vitro lymphocyte responses. Chest, 99(5): 1172-1176.

Heckheimer, E.F. (1989). Health promotion of the elderly in the community. Philadelphia: W.B. Saunders.

Kane, R.L., Ouslander, J.G. & Abrass, I.B.(1984). Essentials of clinical geriatrics. New York: McGraw-Hill.

Mallet, L. (1992). Tuberculin skin test identifies residents with tuberculosis. Provider, 18(8): 47.

Matteson, M.A. & McConnell, E.S. (1988). Gerontological nursing: Concepts and practice. Philadelphia: W.B. Saunders.

Saxon, S.V. & Etten, M.J. (1987). Physical change and aging: A guide for the helping professions (2nd ed.). New York: Tiresias Press.

Staab, A. & Lyles, M. (1990). Manual of geriatric nursing. Glenview, IL: Scott, Foresman & Company.

Stead, W.W. (1991). Tuberculosis control in nursing homes. Choices in Respiratory Management, 21(4): 84-89.

Stead, W.W. (1987). Why does tuberculosis remain so common among the elderly? Hospital Practice, 22(9): 9, 13.

Reproductive

MODULE 7 - *AGE-RELATED CHANGES IN REPRODUCTIVE SYSTEMS AND LATE LIFE SEXUALITY*

Objectives

On completion of this module, the student should be able to:

1. describe normal age-related changes which occur in the reproductive systems of men and women;
2. relate these changes to needs for sexuality among older adults; and
3. apply knowledge about sexuality in later years by developing a plan (with goals and interventions for teaching), and ways of evaluating effectiveness.

Normal age-related changes

Women

Menopause is a physiological process that takes place over three to five years between the early 40s and 50s in which the ovaries reduce their production of female sex hormones. This phase is called the **climacteric** or **perimenopause** and is characterized by physical and emotional changes. Symptoms include irregular menses, hot flashes (sudden sensation of intense heat or flushing usually on the face and neck, and accompanied by sweating), headaches, neckaches, excessive fatigue, feelings of emotional instability, interruption of sleep, irritability, and sometimes depression. Some women experience very few symptoms while others have quite a lot. Cigarette smokers tend to have earlier menopause than nonsmokers. Menopause is considered complete when a woman has been without periods for one year. This ends the ability of the woman to bear children.

The *emotional response* to menopause is affected by individual and cultural factors. If a woman's personal expectations about having children have not been met, the reaction can be poor. For example, if a woman feels that her "biological clock" is running out and she has not had the opportunity to have children, the menopause can be dreaded. Alternately, for the woman who has been pregnant (especially many times), menopause can cause her to feel free, since she will no longer have to worry about becoming pregnant.

In more traditional societies with large family units, the woman's role after her childbearing years is replaced by new and valued roles as a matriarch. In modern youth-orientated societies with more nuclear family structures, the adjustment to her role after the childbearing years may be more difficult. She may have a greater struggle identifying a new role within a small family and within the marriage and society, especially if femininity is associated with fertility. Menopause may also be seen as the onset of aging and approaching death. In more traditional societies where old age and death are considered part of the life cycle, this may pose little anxiety; in modern youth-centered societies, the anxiety may be greater.

As a result of the decline of female hormones especially oestrogen, sex organs, the urinary tract and skin begin to show signs of aging. Up to the point of menopause, female hormones appear to protect women against the risk of heart disease. After menopause, the absence of hormones increases the risk for atherosclerotic plaques. Hormonal decline also causes osteoporosis, resulting in brittle bones and a greater chance of fractures. The breasts become flatter and sag as tissue and mammary ducts atrophy, the vagina becomes less elastic, thinner, narrower and shorter, vaginal secretions are smaller in amount and more watery, and the vaginal pH becomes less alkaline. The cervix and uterus decrease in size, and there is less pubic hair. The labia may become less firm, and the fat pad in the pubic area may lose some of the fatty tissue. Except for the effects of oestrogen loss after menopause, these changes interfere very little with a woman's sexual ability.

IMPLICATIONS AND RECOMMENDATIONS

Hormone replacement therapy (HRT) is the administration of the female hormones oestrogen and progesterone. HRT can be given in several forms such as pills, transdermal patches, and vaginal creams, but each route has different benefits and limitations which must be evaluated individually between each woman and the physician. Also depending on the type of HRT chosen, the woman may begin to have periods once again, or the combination of hormones chosen may not result in new onset of menses.

The benefits of HRT include:

1. HRT oestrogen is protective against heart disease. Oestrogen has been found to *increase high density lipoproteins (HDLs)* which reduce cholesterol in the bloodstream, and to *decrease the low density lipoproteins (LDLs)* which cause fatty deposits on the walls of arteries.
2. HRT offers protection against osteoporosis.
3. HRT eliminates many of the unpleasant symptoms of menopause such as hot flashes.

The risks of HRT are:

1. There is some evidence that oestrogen replacement can lead to development of preexisting oestrogen dependent cancers and noncancerous fibroid tumors in the uterus.
2. HRT may increase the formation of blood clots and hypertension.
3. HRT may lead to breast and endometrial cancers.
4. HRT may cause side effects of fluid retention, breast tenderness, mood changes and other premenstrual-like symptoms (PMS).

Vitamins, herbs and teas have also been suggested as helping to relieve menopausal symptoms. Although they have not been studied extensively. Vitamins E and B_6 have been proposed to reduce hot flashes and fatigue. Ginseng contains compounds that have effects similar to oestrogen. Foods such as alfalfa, cherries, sesame seeds contain plant oestrogens. Hot flashes (which often occur at night) can be made less troublesome by dressing in layers so clothes can be removed as necessary, and drinking liquids at the beginning of a hot flash.

With loss of oestrogen, the usually acid vaginal secretions become less acidic, sometimes causing burning and itching (called **atrophic vaginitis**), and increasing the possibility of vaginal infection. Gynaecological exams including Pap tests should be done at least annually. Symptoms of uncomplicated atrophic vaginitis can subside spontaneously; if symptoms persist, comfort measures such as lubricating creams and gels can be inserted.

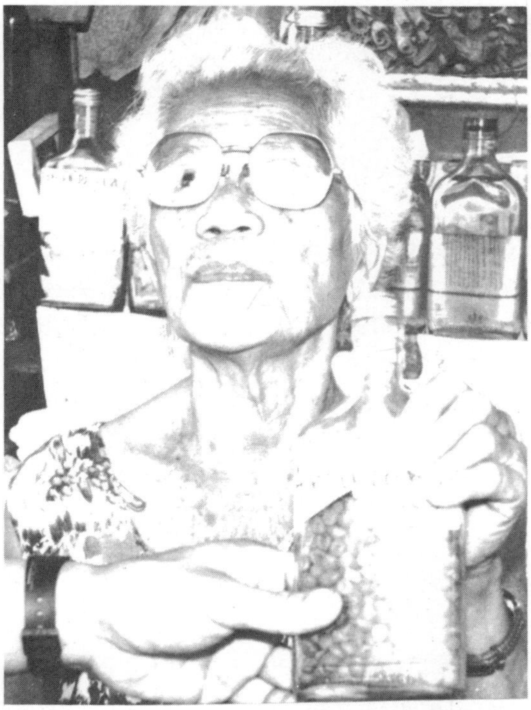

Photo courtesy of T. Miller

This is a picture of herbal products being sold for the elderly in the Philippines. Various herbs and herbal products can harmonize and balance the function of the body. Under certain cultures, many families still keep their own way to prepare herbal teas, decoctions or soft extracts as tonic medicine for age-related changes. In some countries, similar herbal products are available in the market. However, the use of herbal products is based mainly on traditional and cultural beliefs.

Thinner vaginal walls and decreased fat in the pubic area, leave the urethra less protected, and older women may develop **cystitis** (inflammation of the bladder). This requires medical treatment of the infecting organism. Lowered hormone levels also contribute to "stress" or "urge" incontinence. This requires extensive management which is covered in the module on the urinary system.

Men

Older men do not experience hormonal changes to the extent that women do, although testosterone decreases throughout maturity. The main effect is on differences in penile erection. However, the changes which occur have little effect on sexual performance. During sexual intercourse, it takes longer to obtain an erection, the erection may not be as large and hard, ejaculations are smaller in volume, duration and intensity, seminal fluid is thicker, and there is a longer period of time between ejaculations from several hours up to several days. Sperm production generally does not end until the mid-seventies. Most men over 65 years of age have at least some enlargement of the prostate.

Late life sexuality

Sexuality is much more than simply the act of sexual intercourse. It ranges from holding hands, dancing, shared activities and flirting to the act of coitus. Sexuality is a normal and healthy part of life which continues throughout the older years. It is strongly associated with the need for interpersonal relationships, the need for physical and emotional intimacy, the need for love and affection, and one's self-image.

The expression of sexuality is affected by (1) cultural norms, (2) individual and family attitudes, value systems and religious beliefs, (3) physical and emotional health, and (4) environmental factors.

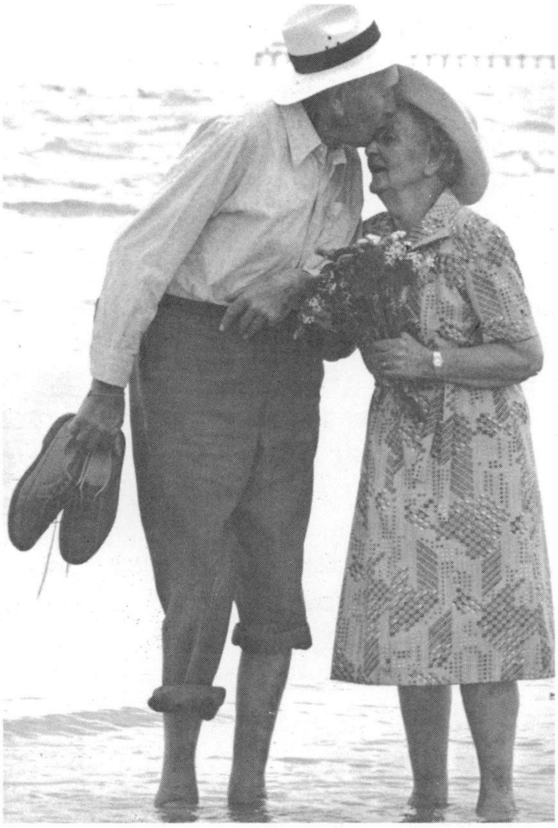

Photo courtesy of Steve Morenos

Sexuality is strongly associated with the need for interpersonal relationships, the need for physical and emotional intimacy, the need for love and affection and one's self-image.

There is much variation among cultures in acceptable and preferred sexual acts, and levels of intimacy between partners (Hotvedt, 1983). All cultures also have myths about sexual practices. For example, it might be believed that (1) older people have no sex drive, or (2) sexual behaviour among older people is not decent. There may also be stereotypes such as describing sexual behaviour in older men as "dirty old men" and in women as "being cute". According to Butler and Lewis (1982; 1993), myths and stereotypes can lead to "ageism", which is discrimination against people because they are old. By denying the needs for sexual expression in the elderly, society makes the aged sexually invisible. Feelings of self-worth and attractiveness are threatened at a time when the need for intimacy and belonging is greatest, and this can lead to loneliness and isolation (Rieve, 1989). As members of society, health care workers also may hold negative views about the sexuality of older adults.

An older person's attitude to sexuality depends in part on his or her past experiences. If an older person had an active and enjoyable sex life and sense of sexuality in the younger years, it is likely that it will be the same in later years. The reverse is also true. Positive psychological development, including the ability to achieve psychological intimacy, reinforces healthy progression in sexual relationships as one ages. However, even with good experiences early on, older people can become the target of negative reactions from family members. This is especially true if an older person goes to live with his or her children. Sons and daughters are sometimes uncomfortable and not accepting of the sexuality of their elderly parents.

Physical health problems including cardiovascular and respiratory diseases, cancer, arthritis, osteoporosis, neurological disorders such as Parkinson's disease, anemia, and functional limitations can reduce sexual desire and activity. In *men*, chronic prostatitis and diabetes, especially if not well controlled, may be particular concerns. In *women,* chronic cystitis and stress or urge incontinence are frequent problems in sexual activity. As in all age groups, any surgery which greatly affects physical appearance (such as mastectomy or colostomy) can cause doubt about self-image and attractiveness to the partner. Counselling before and after surgery, support groups, prosthetic devices, and cosmetic concealments are indicated.

Again, as in all age groups, sexually transmitted diseases (STDs) pose a very difficult situation. Syphilis is one type. Both partners need testing. If the results are positive, there may be loss of trust by the partner who gets infected, since the originally-infected partner was probably not monogamous or possibly violated cultural taboos (Butler & Lewis). Syphilis is not infectious after it has been present for five years or longer (Butler & Lewis, 1993). Recently AIDS has become a serious STD as well, and carries with it the real danger of life-threatening illness. Gonorrhoea and other forms of STDs should also be considered in assessments.

The emotional state of the older person affects sexual performance. Grief over death of loved ones, role adjustment post menopause and/or following retirement, fear, stress and worry, lack of privacy when living with children or when living in a nursing home or other institutional setting all interfere with feelings of sexuality. The death of a lifelong partner may leave the remaining person frustrated.

Many drugs have side effects which either reduce sexual desire or cause impotency (in men). Sedatives, certain pain medications, antispasmodics, tranquilizers, antidepressants and certain medications used to control high blood pressure can impair male erection. Their effects on women are less well understood. Most drugs can be adjusted by the physician to reduce symptoms. Alcohol is a drug and a depressant. In large amounts it interferes with sexual performance. Tolerance for alcohol also decreases with age and alcohol is dangerous in combination with medications.

IMPLICATIONS AND RECOMMENDATIONS

In counselling older persons who seek advice, health care workers should (1) emphasize the **quality** of relationships with a focus on the *person* rather than the *performance*, and (2) be well informed and comfortable with their own sexuality so that correct, unbiased information is provided (Weg, 1983). Sexuality should always be described in the broadest sense (that is beyond just sexual intercourse) including social participation, finding meaning in relationships, holding hands, hugging and so on.

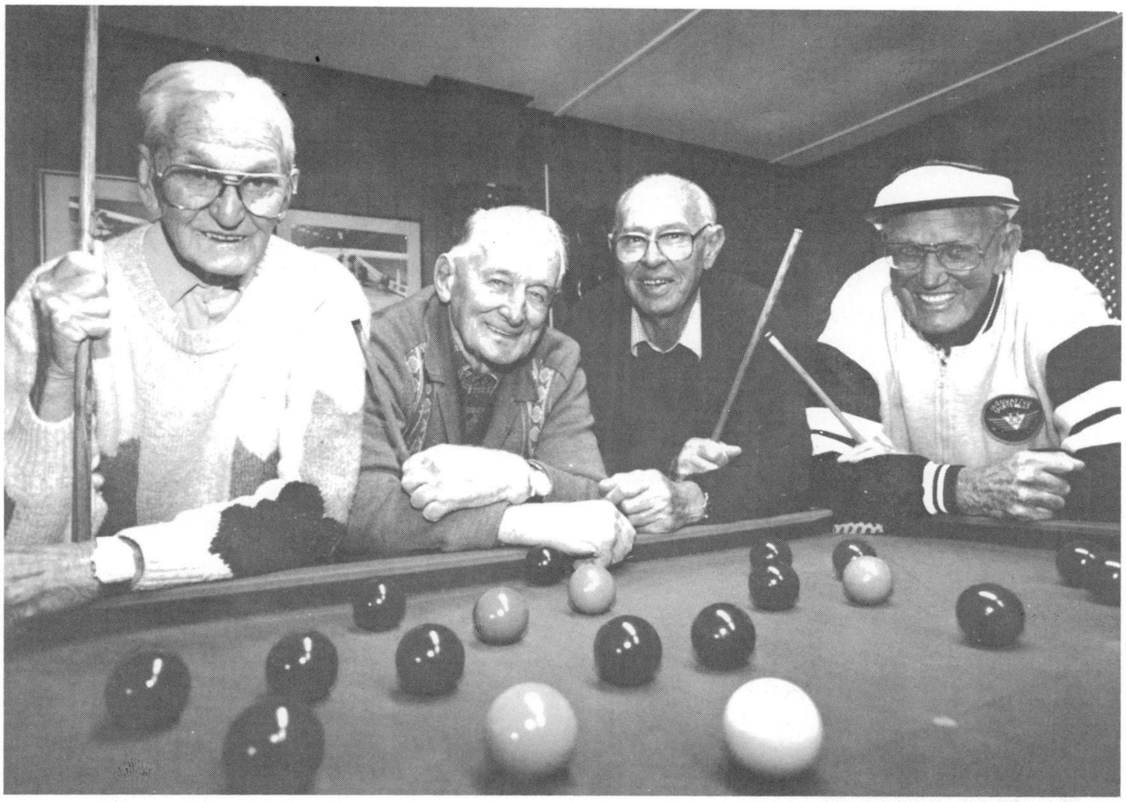

Photo courtesy of Peter Morgan

These elderly mates "just enjoy themselves". Counselling older persons should focus on the quality of relationships and not the performance.

Carefully worded assessment questions can help older people feel comfortable talking about sexuality. Examples include: "Does your present health interfere in any way with your sexual function?", "Is there anything about your sexual activity that you would like to change?", "Is there anything you would like to ask about sexual intimacy?" Women might prefer to discuss these things with females and men with male health care workers.

The nurse may need to act as facilitator with the older person's adult children, discussing the need for privacy, suggesting ways in which privacy might be arranged, and helping with the adult children's reactions to dating or remarrying. Educating the family of the older person is an important step in changing negative attitudes and stereotypes. In addition to the adult children, and as the occasion arises naturally, grandchildren should be sensitively taught about sexuality in simple ways such as using the correct anatomical terms in referring to body parts and functions. Recommendations should not put the family in conflict with their cultural or religious values.

For those with chronic illnesses, the partners may need more in-depth assessment about their sexuality prior to the onset of the disability, and more adaptation of interventions. Chronic illness does not have to result in loss of sexual intimacy. Maintaining sexual behaviours, especially ones such as touching, holding, kissing, and talking, helps the partner retain that relationship rather than becoming solely a caregiver. In these situations, cleanliness and hygiene, care of appliances such as catheters, Kegel exercises for incontinence management and so on are particularly important.

It is always important to feel attractive and look one's best. This includes no smoking, moderate use of alcohol, control of blood pressure and weight, balanced nutrition, regular exercise, attention to personal appearance and use of fragrances and other cosmetic pleasantries as desired. Age-related physical changes in the reproductive and musculoskeletal systems can be easily managed by small adjustments, for example (1) using side-lying positions for sexual intercourse, (2) applying water soluble lubricants help moisten the mucous membranes of the vagina, and (3) taking warm showers or baths to ease arthritis.

Exercise A

Enact the following situation in a role-play. Mrs. R has come to the health centre because of vaginal dryness. She has been told by a friend that this can be a sign of aging. In addition to the vaginal dryness, she now hardly ever experiences a menstrual period. Have one student play the part of the health care worker and take a sexual history. Let another student play the part of Mrs. R. The group then analyses whether the interview questions were *sensitively* worded, and gives examples. Is Mrs. R completely menopausal or is she perimenopausal? What suggestions and information can be given to help her?

Exercise B

As a group, explore your own feelings about sexuality and analyse how these may influence your ability to counsel and advise older persons on this topic. Does it embarrass you to discuss sexuality? What are acceptable behaviours and what are taboos in your culture?

Short-answer exercise

1. Briefly describe the physiological changes which take place in female menopause.

2. What are some of the concerns about privacy when older parents live with their adult children?

Bibliography

Ackermann, U. (1992). Essentials of human physiology. St. Louis: Mosby Year Book.

Butler, R.N. & Lewis, M.I. (1993). Love and sex after 60. New York: Ballantine Books.

Datan, N. & Rodeheaver, D. (1983). Beyond generativity: Toward a sensuality of later life. In R.B. Weg (Ed.) Sexuality in the later years: Roles and behaviour, (pp. 279-288), New York: Academic Press.

Dressel, P.L. & Avant, R. (1983). Range of alternatives. In R.B. Weg (Ed.) Sexuality in the later years: Roles and behavior, (pp. 185-207), New York: Academic Press.

Glass, J.C. & Dalton, J.A. (1988). Sexuality in older adults: A continuing education concern. The Journal of Continuing Education in Nursing, 19(2): 61-64.

Hite, S. (1976). The Hite report. New York: MacMillan Publishing Company.

Hotvedt, M. (1983). The cross-cultural and historical context. In R.B. Weg (Ed.) Sexuality in the later years: Roles and behavior, (pp. 13-37), New York: Academic Press.

Landau, E. & Maoz, B. (1983). Continuity of self-actualization: Womanhood in the climacterium and old age. In R.B. Weg (Ed.) Sexuality in the later years: Roles and behavior, (pp. 251-258), New York: Academic Press.

McCracken, A.L. (19?). Sexual practice by elders: The forgotten aspect of functional health. Journal of Gerontological Nursing, 14(10): 13-17.

Kim, M.J. (Ed.)(1993). Primary health care: Nurses lead the way-A global perspective (Case studies of WHO collaborating centres for nursing/midwifery development). American Association of Colleges of Nursing (ISBN 0-922148-06-6)

Mooradian, A.D. (1991). Geriatric sexuality and chronic diseases, Geriatric Sexuality, 7(1): 113-131.

National Institute on Aging (December 1992). Menopause. National Institutes of Health (United States Government Printing Office Publication No. ISBN 0-16-038139-8). Washington, DC: US GPO.

Rieve, J.E. (1989). Sexuality and the adult with acquired physical disability. Nursing Clinics of North America, 24(1): 265-276.

Roughan, P.A., Kaiser, F.E. & Morley, J.E. (1993). Sexuality and the older woman. Clinics in Geriatric Medicine, 9(1): 87-106.

Smedley, G. (1991). Addressing sexuality in the elderly. Rehabilitation Nursing, 16(1): 9-11.

Weg, R.B. (Ed.)(1983). Sexuality in the later years: Roles and behavior. New York: Academic Press.

White, C.B. & Catania, J.A. (1982). Psychoeducational intervention for sexuality with the aged, family members of the aged, and people who work with the aged. International Journal of Human Aging & Human Development, 15(2): 121-138.

Winn, R.I. & Newton, N. (1982). Sexuality in aging: A study of 106 cultures. Archives of Sexual Behavior, 11(4): 283-298.

Zeiss, R.A., Delmonico, R.L., Zeiss, A.M. & Dornbrand, L. (1991). Psychologic disorder and sexual dysfunction in elders. Geriatric Sexuality, 7(1): 133-151.

Endocrine and Immune Function

MODULE 8 - *ENDOCRINE AND IMMUNE FUNCTION*

Objectives

On completion of this module, the student should be able to:

1. describe (selected) normal age-related changes which occur in endocrine and immune function; and
2. apply knowledge about non-insulin dependent diabetes mellitus (NIDDM) by developing a plan (with goals and interventions for teaching) for the disease, and ways of evaluating effectiveness.

Normal age-related changes

Endocrine system

As one gets older, the weight of the thyroid gland decreases and there is more connective tissue and less colloid. The basal metabolic rate (BMR) is lower due to reduction in the mass of functioning cells, rather than to a decrease in their metabolic activity. However, the rate is still adequate for normal functioning of older persons.

There is **decreased** secretion of the antidiuretic hormone (ADH) as described in Module 4.

The changes in insulin are not yet fully understood nor fully explained. There is a slight decline in insulin as one gets older, a slower and more prolonged release of insulin, a decrease in receptor sites for the insulin-glucose interaction, and decreased reabsorption of glucose in the renal tubules.

Immune function

Immune function is a very complicated aspect of physiology, and again, changes in immune function are not conclusive. The immune response functions to protect the body from invading organisms. In general, it appears that immune function declines with age. There is a *reduction in response to antigens*. For example, older people have a delayed response to testing using purified protein derivative (PPD) for tuberculosis. There is some evidence that *natural antibodies are decreased, autoantibodies are increased, and cytotoxic T cells are fewer.*

Some support for these findings may be demonstrated in the increased tendency for **pneumonia** among older people, and the increase in the **rate of cancer** as age increases.

IMPLICATIONS

Less effective ADH function causes older persons to lose more water than younger persons. Excessive heat, diarrhoea, vomiting and diuretics can accelerate the process and the danger of electrolyte loss and cardiac irregularities.

REMEMBER: *Confusion is often the first sign of dehydration and sodium loss in older people.*

Alteration in insulin and immune function result in a slower, less effective response to stress. Any challenge to the system such as excessive physical activity or infection, can cause older persons to become weakened and less independent.

Illnesses

Diabetes Mellitus is actually a category of illness, rather than a single disease, in which several disorders are characterized by glucose intolerance. There are two major classifications: insulin dependent diabetes mellitus (IDDM) or Type I diabetes and non-insulin dependent diabetes mellitus (NIDDM) or Type II diabetes.

There is a reduction in the biological effectiveness of insulin as one ages. Almost half of all persons over 65 years of age have either impaired glucose tolerance or diabetes mellitus (Minaker, 1990). NIDDM is the most common type of diabetes in older persons. Unlike IDDM where there is a lack of insulin produced, in older persons there are fewer receptor sites available for binding of insulin and glucose. For this reason, although there is only a slight decline in glucose production, there is a *relative* insulin deficiency because of the poor uptake of glucose. The poor uptake of insulin impairs the metabolism of carbohydrates, proteins and fats, tissue breakdown occurs and results in chronic complications of the cardiovascular system, retina, renal glomeruli, and nervous system (peripheral neuropathy).

In older people, NIDDM is often found by chance in the course of a routine examination or during the search for the cause of other problems such as visual disturbance, chronic skin infections, delayed healing of skin lesions, urinary or vaginal infections, or complaints of numbness in the leg.

It is found by chance, in part because the symptoms are often vague and subtle, and can mimic other normal age-related changes. Symptoms include thirst, fatigue, subtle mental changes, weight loss, blurred vision, muscle weakness, itching without a rash, and sugar in the urine. The presence of sugar in the urine is highly suggestive of diabetes in older persons because they have an increased normal renal threshold *meaning* that they should be less likely to have sugar in their urine.

Factors which contribute to NIDDM include living a sedentary lifestyle and being overweight.

Interventions are aimed at two goals:

1. accomplishing changes in behaviour to increase reasonable exercise and reduce weight through diet management; and

2. minimizing the complications of diabetes including loss of vision and infection and loss of feet and legs, through education of the older person and the family.

Oral hypoglycemic agents are the primary treatment for older persons when diet and exercise do not control blood sugar levels.

REMEMBER:	**to incorporate knowledge about age-related changes into education and management of diabetes control. For example, dipsticks require colour matching of strips to a chart. The strips and charts are very small and the blue and green shades are precisely the colours that older people see less well. Handling the paper strips requires a fair amount of fine motor coordination and dexterity. Family members may need to do the test and interpret the results for the older person.**

As another example, difficulties with chewing might need to be solved in order to achieve dietary goals.

Since visual problems are one of the greatest problems associated with diabetes, eye exams should be done regularly.

Leg and feet problems are common and are due to neurological and vascular changes. Injuries to these extremities are slower to heal, more readily infected and harder to treat with systemic antibiotics. Infections which progress to loss of feet and legs greatly increase the likelihood that the older person will lose mobility and independence. It is vital that they be protected from injury and infection.

Atherosclerosis, arteriosclerosis and hypertension are increased in older adults with diabetes. Coronary deaths account for half the deaths of people with NIDDM.

Exercise

If a clinical field experience is NOT planned, a case study can be proposed and a plan of care developed by the group.

Short-answer exercise

Describe how insulin uptake is different for older people. They are not actually deficient in insulin.

Suggested field experience for assessment of practical skills

Students can be assigned to a health care centre or community where they can have a chance to work with older persons who have non-insulin dependent diabetes mellitus. Select older people with interesting needs and have students develop a complete plan of care.

Bibliography

Brookbank, J.W.(1990). The biology of aging. New York: Harper & Row.

Brown, S.A. (1990). Studies of educational interventions and outcomes in diabetic adults: A meta-analysis revisited. Patient Education Consultant, 16(3): 189-215.

Carnevali, D.L. & Patrick, M. (Eds.)(1993). Nursing management for the elderly (3rd ed.). Philadelphia: J.B. Lippincott.

Christensen, M.H., Funnell, M.M., Ehrlich, M.R., Fellows, E.P., & Floyd, J.C. (1991). How to care for the diabetic foot. American Journal of Nursing. 91(3): 50-56.

Gilden, J.L., Hendryx, M., Casia, C., & Singh, S.P. (1989). The effectiveness of diabetes education programs for older patients and their spouses. Journal of American Geriatrics Society, 37(11): 1023-1030.

Greenspan, F.S. & Baxter, J.D. (Eds.)(1994). Basic & clinical endocrinology (4th ed.). Norwalk, CN: Appleton & Lange.

Hampton, J.K. (1991). The biology of human aging. Dubuque, IA: Wm. C. Brown.

Harris, M.J. (1992). Onset of NIDDM occurs at least 4-7 years before clinical diagnosis. Diabetes Care, 15(7): 815-819.

Heckheimer, E.F. (1989). Health promotion of the elderly in the community. Philadelphia: W.B. Saunders.

Henry, R.R., & Edelman, S.V. (1992). Advances in type II diabetes mellitus in the elderly. Geriatrics, 47(4): 24-30.

Kane, R.L., Ouslander, J.G. & Abrass, I.B.(1984). Essentials of clinical geriatrics. New York: McGraw-Hill.

Lipsky, B.A. (1991). Diabetic foot infections: Pathophysiology, diagnosis and treatment. International Journal of Dermatology, 30(8): 560-562.

Matteson, M.A. & McConnell, E.S. (1988). Gerontological nursing: Concepts and practice. Philadelphia: W.B. Saunders.

Mason, J.E., Rimm, E.B., & Stampfer. (1992). Physical activity and incidence of non-insulin-dependent diabetes mellitus in women. Lancet, 338(8770): 774-728.

Minaker, K. (1990). What diabetologists should know about elderly patients. Diabetes Care 13 (supplement): 2.

Saxon, S.V. & Etten, M.J. (1987). Physical change and aging: A guide for the helping professions (2nd ed.). New York: Tiresias Press.

Staab, A. & Lyles, M. (1990). Manual of geriatric nursing. Glenview, IL: Scott, Foresman & Company.

Dementing Illness

MODULE 9 - *DEMENTING ILLNESS AND CHANGES IN THE BRAIN*

Objectives

On completion of this module, the student should be able to:

1. explain age-related changes which occur in the brain;
2. describe current explanations for the cause and progression of Alzheimer's disease; and
3. apply knowledge about dementia by developing a plan (with goals and interventions) for older persons with this problem, and ways of evaluating effectiveness.

Normal age-related changes in the brain

The changes in the brain are numerous and a comprehensive description of them is beyond the scope of this module. In brief, there is a loss of brain cells, the brain becomes smaller and the ventricles (which contain the fluid) enlarge. Lipofuscin (a brownish pigment in nerve cells) and plaque, including amyloid, accumulate. There is also some reduced transmission efficiency (that is communication among brain cells), probably due to the smaller number of cells. *These changes seem to have no real functional significance since the normal older brain is still quite capable of learning and remembering*. In cases where normal age-related changes have been found in diseases of the brain, for example the accumulation of plaque in Alzheimer's disease, the disease seems to occur because the amount of the substance present is excessive.

Dementia

In this module, the major category of illness described which affects the brain of older persons is dementia.

Dementia is a disturbance in mental processing which is characterized by:

- impaired short-term and long-term memory, and
- impaired abstract thinking and judgement.

There are two major classifications of dementia, **acute** (also known as **reversible** dementia) and **chronic** (also termed **nonreversible** dementia).

Acute or reversible dementia has an abrupt or sudden onset. In other words, the beginning of the confusional state can be reasonably well traced to a specific point or period of time, when there was a clear and distinct change in behaviour. This type of dementia is generally due to one of the following:

- the side effects of medications;
- electrolyte imbalance, especially low sodium (hyponatremia) and dehydration;
- nutritional deficiencies;
- diseases, especially those associated with oxygen deficiency such as anaemia, hypotension and altered blood sugar (hypo or hyperglycaemia);
- urinary tract infections and pneumonia;
- changes in body temperature (hypothermia and hyperthermia);

- depression;
- deficiencies in hearing or vision which cause confusion in understanding and responding appropriately, and
- relocation to unfamiliar places and people.

Acute dementia can be resolved by correcting the underlying cause. Hence, it is termed reversible. The causes of dementia listed above should always be explored first, in order to be certain that the confusion is not temporary and correctable.

Chronic dementia has an onset which cannot usually be traced to a known period. In fact, the symptoms are usually extremely subtle and gradual, and progress over an extended period of time. *The course of the disease is one of gradual but inevitable decline*. Hence, it is termed irreversible. The disturbance in thinking, reasoning, judgement and memory significantly interfere with the older persons' daily activities and interpersonal relationships.

Among the forms of chronic dementia are (1) the Alzheimer's type, (2) multi-infarct dementia, or dementia due to stroke or cardiovascular disease, (3) dementia of totally unknown cause, or (4) a combination of any of these. It is not possible to conclusively diagnose the form of dementia except by autopsy. However, the Alzheimer's type is clearly the most catastrophic for the older person and the family.

Most recent work on Alzheimer's disease (AD) has centered on the discovery of proteins or other molecules that can be linked to the disease. Alzheimer's disease is characterized by the presence in the brain of **senile plaques** (formed from broken parts of neurons, the centre of the plaque accumulates an abnormal protein and the plaque interferes with the ability of the neurons to send and receive messages), **neurofibrillary tangles** (twisted fibres that accumulate inside the body of a neuron), death of large number of **neurons** resulting in shrinkage of the brain, and changes in **neurotransmitters** (the chemicals needed by cells to transmit signals).

There is evidence that **chromosome 21** (the same one on which Down's syndrome is found) is associated with **early onset** AD (begins at a younger than expected age), while **chromosome 19** is associated with the more typical **late onset** form of the disease.

For late onset AD, it has been found that a variation of a gene on chromosome 19, is more common in persons with AD. *The gene is called* ***ApoE*** and seems to be involved with growth and repair of cells in the nervous system by maintaining the cell membrane and preventing damage to nerve tracts. ApoE proteins appear to be present in neurofibrillary tangles and this has led to speculation that different versions of ApoE interact with other substances in the body, such as proteins in senile plaques and neurofibrillary tangles, causing brain cells to disintegrate. *There are several versions of the blood protein ApoE*. They are ApoE-2, ApoE-3 and ApoE-4.

Most people are born with ApoE-3. But most AD patients appear to have ApoE-4 rather than E-3.

The ApoE-3 regulates phosphate in the brain and prevents it from destroying critical nerve tracts. Too much phosphorous leads to the formation of neurofibrillary tangles. In persons with AD, the plaque in the brain contains an insoluble sticky material called beta amyloid to which ApoE-4 is attached. Researchers speculate that it is *not* the presence of **ApoE-4** that *causes* the disease, rather it is the *absence* of **ApoE-3** to keep nerves in the brain alive.

It is not known why, but about 25% of AD victims develop Parkinson's disease and vice versa.

Many pharmacological approaches are being examined. Hydergine, a recent test drug, has been found to be *ineffective* in improving the mental abilities of persons with AD. Desferal is another experimental drug currently being studied, and there is speculation that anti-inflammatory drugs such as aspirin may assist in the prevention of AD.

Recognizing symptoms, managing behaviour and maintaining function

In the *very early stages of the disease*, the older person may only appear irritable or occasionally *forgetful* or *inattentive*. *Personality changes* are slight. They may seem eccentric but certainly not odd or sick. For example, they may dress differently than before, wear clothes which don't match well, are for the wrong season or occasion, flashy, or in some way quite different from their previous taste and style. Personal hygiene may deteriorate. Hair frequently needs to be combed or washed, clothing is soiled and body odours may be present.

Persons who never used foul language or who never swore in the past may start to do so. They may begin to have overdue bills because they cannot remember to make payments or cannot calculate money any longer. Their *judgement is poor*. For example, they may let strangers into the home. **Depression** may be associated with the early phase of the disease while there is enough orientation remaining for persons to know that something is happening to their mind.

The initial stage lasts from about two to four years, although the different stages overlap. As the older person deteriorates, more functions are affected and problem behaviours increase. Among the *functions* affected by dementia and which show a decline are:

- ability to pay attention;
- verbal skills (language and the ability to communicate);

- social skills;
- higher cognition (intellectual functioning);
- numerical skills (adding, subtracting etc.);
- abstraction;
- recognition (of familiar faces and objects); and
- memory (short-term and long-term).

Behavioural problems which increase as the disease progresses may include:

- wandering away and/or wandering about during the night;
- incontinence of urine and stool and possibly smearing bowel products;
- delusions and hallucinations;
- suspicion and hostility which causes aggressive behaviour (hitting, screaming, biting); and
- taking clothes off inappropriately.

In the *later stages of the disease,* people lose the ability to dress, bathe, feed and toilet themselves, and eventually they become totally dependent on others. Older people can live for many years with dementia. The disease progresses slowly for five to ten years after the initial changes.

IMPLICATIONS AND RECOMMENDATIONS

The degree of impairment from the disease can be assessed by asking simple questions. For example, one can ask the day of the week, the month, the year, who is the current head of state, what was eaten for breakfast, to add or subtract numbers, and recognition of simple objects such as coins and fruits. Responses will give an indication of the mental ability for recent and remote (past) memory, and intellectual performance.

> In all situations, the major objectives are: (1) *protecting* the demented person from harm, (2) *maintaining independence in daily activities* as long as possible, (3) *improving communication*, (4) *preventing* and/or *reducing the occurrence* of difficult behaviours and (5) providing *support to family caregivers.*

(1) Many things in the home must be considered in planning for *safety*. If the demented person turns the stove on, then fire is a potential hazard.

If the stove is electric, it should be disconnected when the elderly is at home alone as well as during the night if they wander throughout the house. If wandering away from the home is a problem, the older person must always be under someone's observation in order to be secured and protected. The most important point is to *anticipate* the safety needs by conducting a thorough assessment of risk.

(2) In order to maintain *independence* as long as possible, demented persons must be kept stimulated and involved in activities.

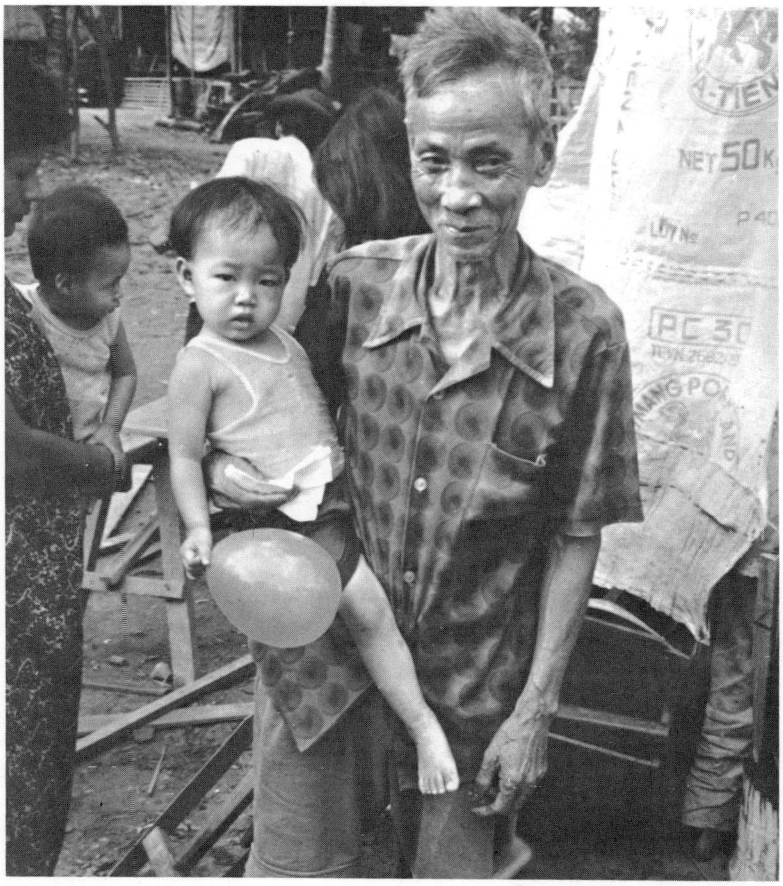

Photo courtesy of Dr. Bilous

Older adults can stay active and involved by sharing their wisdom and experience. In Viet Nam, the elderly are a valuable human resource. In this photo the grandfather cares for the grandchild while the parents are away from home working.

Reality Orientation (RO) is one approach which is simple, can be done by health care workers and families, can be done while other daily activities are being carried out, and can be done in any setting. *In order to be most effective, RO should be carried out in two ways*: through the use of groups and throughout the day and evening on a one-to-one basis.

In regard to the group method, meetings should be held (a) by two people co-leading for two weeks (ideally) in a row in order to give *continuity*, (b) at the same time and place each day to provide *predictability*, and (c) for about

30-minute sessions daily *to avoid fatigue* of older persons. The group size should be limited from four to six *members so that plenty of individual attention* can be given. Pictures of well known places such as churches and animals, photographs of friends, family and pets, items for gardening, and so on can be used to remind elderly about facts associated with these things.

The process of RO should also be continued throughout the hours when awake. RO boards should be displayed which contain information which helps orientate demented persons to current weather conditions, day of the week, month and year, holidays and many other points of daily living. *Remember to keep the board up-to-date.*

Throughout the day, if the older person says something which is confused, such as calling an apple an orange, gently provide correct information by stating, "This is an apple". If the person expresses fear from perceptual distortion, such as believing a broom to be a sword, again clarify by saying, "There is no need to be afraid, see, it is only a broom".

Sensory Stimulation is another approach which is easily incorporated into daily routines and can be done in groups or one-to-one. Select items which can be used to stimulate the senses. For the sense of smell, (a) use things with strong odours/scents such as tea, coffee, flowers, perfumes, cloves, citrus fruits, (b) have the person identify the scent and assist them to recall it as necessary, (c), and talk about the scent, reminding them of its use or an occasion in which it is used. For the sense of touch, (a) select items with different textures such as feathers, cotton balls, wool, linen, silk, (b) have the person identify the item and assist them to recall it as necessary, and (c) develop a theme which can remind them of its use or an occasion in which it is used. Similar things can be done for vision (using bright colours), and for hearing by using things which make different sounds.

Although **communicating** with demented older persons *can be very frustrating*, it is important that health care workers and family caregivers *do not* respond by ignoring the older person, talking to them as if they were a child, answering for the older person before giving them a chance to answer for themselves, or shouting or speaking harshly to the older person.

Instead, communication should stress the following:

- Don't hurry the older person when trying to speak; allow them time to consider what they want to say.
- If the older person starts to forget what they are trying to say, repeat the last words or sentence that they spoke.
- Use short simple sentences and ones which can be answered by a yes or no such as, "Are you comfortable?" or "Did you have enough to eat?"

- Give the most important content of what needs to be communicated at the end of the sentence. For example, "Do you want to have tea or coffee?" *rather than*, "Do you want tea or coffee with your breakfast?"

- When giving instructions, give each direction one at a time. For example, if the older person is toileting, it might be (1) 'Lift your dress up.'; (2) 'Sit down.'; (3) 'Here is the toilet paper.'; (4) 'Wipe yourself.', and so on.

- Reduce background noise and distractions; if possible, take the older person to a quiet place when important messages need to be conveyed.

(4) Part of the importance of *communicating well* and *patiently*, is that this often prevents the occurrence of *agitation* and *other disruptive behaviours.* The most common behaviour problems in AD persons include:

- resisting care and direction;
- screaming;
- repeating things over and over;
- striking out physically;
- inappropriate sexual behaviour;
- taking clothes off in inappropriate places or undressing throughout the day;
- hoarding things; and
- smearing bowel movements.

Observe the elderly and also *interview* family members to determine which factors seem to trigger inappropriate behaviours. Bathing and toileting are common ones which start these behaviours in persons with AD. *Other factors which cause* these behaviours are:

- *too much stimulation* in the environment from people and noise;
- *unfamiliar persons and places*;
- *being forced* to do something;
- *too many instructions* at once;

- *accumulation of physical energy* from inadequate activity and exercise;
- *fatigue, physical discomfort* from pain, fever or constipation; and
- *inability to communicate needs* (frustration).

Sometimes 'touch' can help make the older person feel safe, but at other times it may agitate them. Identify residence and family behaviour situations which need a specific plan of care/management. Describe the feelings and reactions which these behaviour situations evoke in family caregivers.

NOTE:	**Interventions for the older person depend on the self care level and nature of problem behaviours of the person with the dementia.**

Approaches may include the following:

- make a *routine for daily* care including bathing and eating, to improve predictability, thereby giving a sense of security;
- determine the best time of day for doing needed things;
- try not to surprise the person when approaching the care; always say what you are about to do before doing it;
- avoid arguing and physically restraining the person if agitated behaviour begins;
- redirect the person's attention, gently steer them to another focus or leave the issue and try again later;
- be creative and patient with yourself and with the older person; what works one time might not work another time; and
- engage the older person in recreational activities which use the whole body, such as tossing a large soft ball back and forth, group dancing or bending and stretching exercises.

Problems with personal hygiene and odours all need to be dealt with individually, depending on the older person, stage of dementia, and family preferences for interventions.

(5) The *family needs a great deal of emotional support* in taking care of a relative with dementia. This may include coordination with support groups. The family also needs to have arrangements for relief of responsibilities so that the caretaker(s) do not become exhausted and/or socially isolated.

NOTE: **Module 11 "Supporting Families in Caregiving" contains more specific information about helping families.**

Exercise A

Enact the following situation in a role-play. Mrs. P has a 68-year old husband of many years, who has started becoming very forgetful. She tells you that she didn't seek help before for two reasons. First, she thought his loss of memory was just part of his getting old. Second, she said it was very hard to tell whether he was really changing or not. She cannot tell you precisely when it all began, but recently he appears depressed and lacking energy all the time. He used to be an engineer before he retired. Develop the plan including explanation to his wife of normal age-related changes, behaviour management strategies, and emotional support. What stage of the disease do you think he is at?

Exercise B

Divide the students into two groups. Have one group develop everything they would need (including topics and props) to conduct a reality orientation group. Have the other group develop everything they would need to conduct a sensory stimulation group. Be specific in how these activities for the elderly would be carried out. Share the details and ideas with one another.

Short-answer exercise

Briefly describe how acute or reversible dementia differs from chronic or nonreversible dementia.

Suggested field of experience for assessment of practical skills

Students can be assigned to a health care centre where they will have a chance to work with older persons who have dementia problems. If the older persons have no family, perhaps a nursing home would be appropriate. Select an older person and have the students develop a complete plan of care.

Mental Health

MODULE 10 - *MENTAL HEALTH AND AGING*

Objectives

On completion of this module, the student should be able to:

1. describe (selected) influences of cultural background on the provision of mental health support to older adults and their families;

2. identify the most common mental health problems of older adults;

3. apply knowledge about depression by developing a care plan (with goals and interventions) and ways for evaluating the effectiveness; and

4. summarize information about group strategies which are most frequently used to maintain and/or restore the emotional well-being of older persons.

Mental health and aging

A positive mental outlook is essential to healthy aging. However, many issues faced in later years create serious emotional challenges for the elderly.

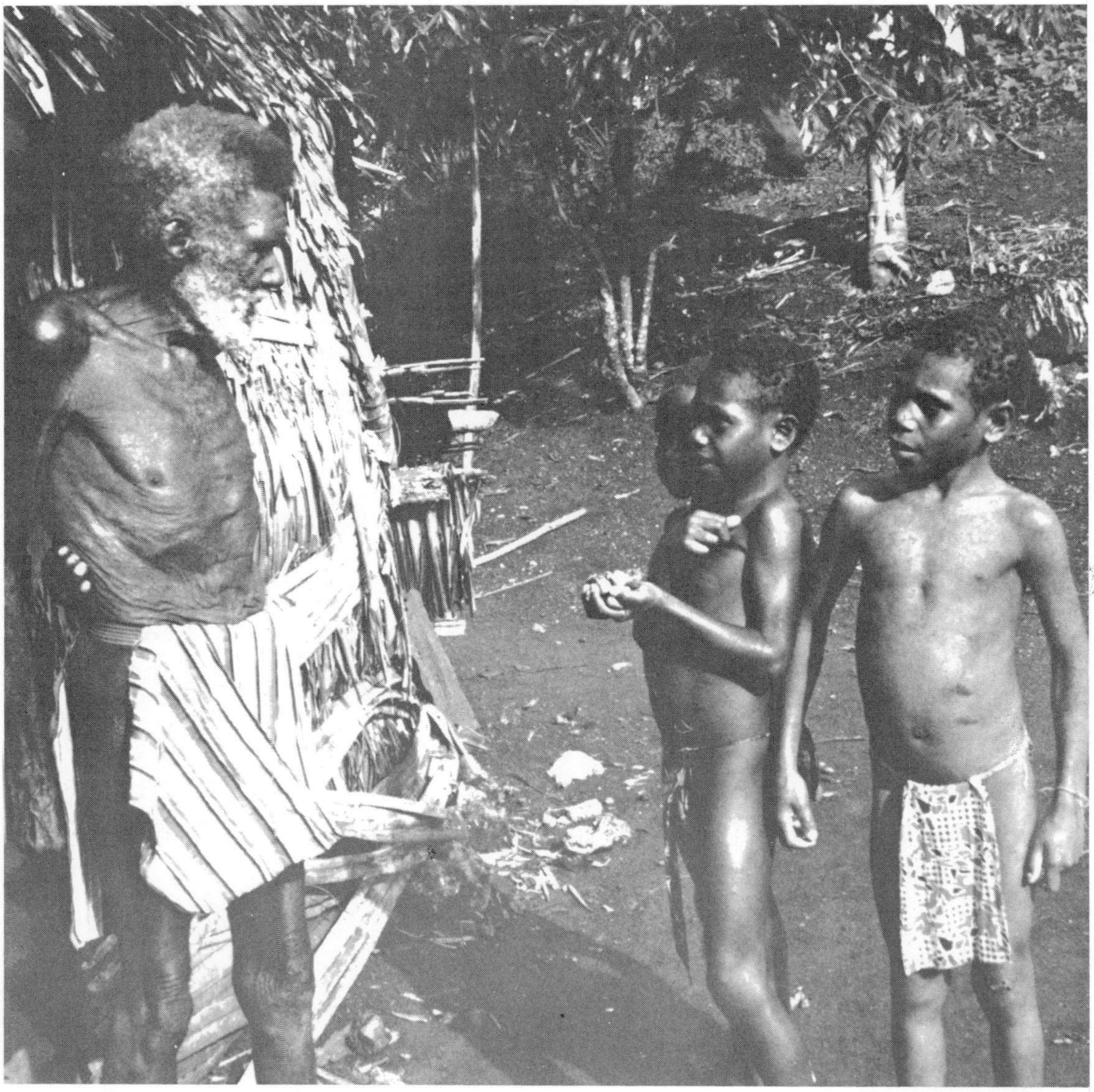

Photo courtesy of T. Miller

Elderly in Vanuatu enjoy, and for the most part add vital knowledge to, the life of the community. They are surrounded with youth who approach them for their ideas. Thus, an active mind and body is fully respected and provides meaningful and satisfying living for the older person.

> **Cultural background** greatly influences *the ways in which older persons cope*, the *willingness* of the elderly and their families *to acknowledge the need for mental health interventions*, and the *willingness* of older persons and their families to seek and accept mental health services.

Older adults and their families may *deny* the existence of mental health problems because:

- they feel these problems are shameful;
- they believe the problem is a repayment for bad deeds;
- they are convinced the healing of illnesses (including emotional ones) is in God's hands;
- they think suffering should be endured;
- they want to appear in control in order to maintain their dignity; and/or
- emotional control is valued in the society and admitting the need for help suggests that one is not in control.

Often, instead of requesting assistance for psychological difficulties, they will seek medical care for **somatic illnesses** such as *headaches*, *insomnia*, *dizziness* or other *vague physical complaints*. They may previously have sought relief from traditional (medicine) healers, especially in cultures where illness is strongly viewed as an imbalance in forces, and the psyche and body are inseparable.

For these reasons, the number of older people in need of mental health support may be greatly underestimated.

Among the most common mental health problems of older adults are:

- *widowhood* and the *deaths of significant others*;
- caregiver *stress*;
- *fears* (of such things as death; financial difficulties associated with retirement, and loss of independence);
- changes from previous roles; and living arrangements; and
- and social isolation.

The emotional response to these problems include **grief, guilt, loneliness, loss of meaning in life and lack of motivation, anxiety, anger, feelings of powerlessness, and depression.**

In addition to individual psychiatric and psychological counselling, group therapy can be effective in promoting good mental health. Among the most frequently used are small *group strategies* of (1) *Remotivation*, (2) *Reminiscence*, (3) *Music*, *Art*, and *Poetry*, (4) *groups for those who are mourning*, and (5) *groups for family members*. Group work with old-age groups requires some special skills. Group leaders typically must provide a great deal of *emotional support* and *encouragement*, help discover sources of *hope and motivation*, focus on *problem solving*, *stress management* and *coping strategies* and manage *functional* and *physical disabilities* and *sensory deficits* of the elderly as well.

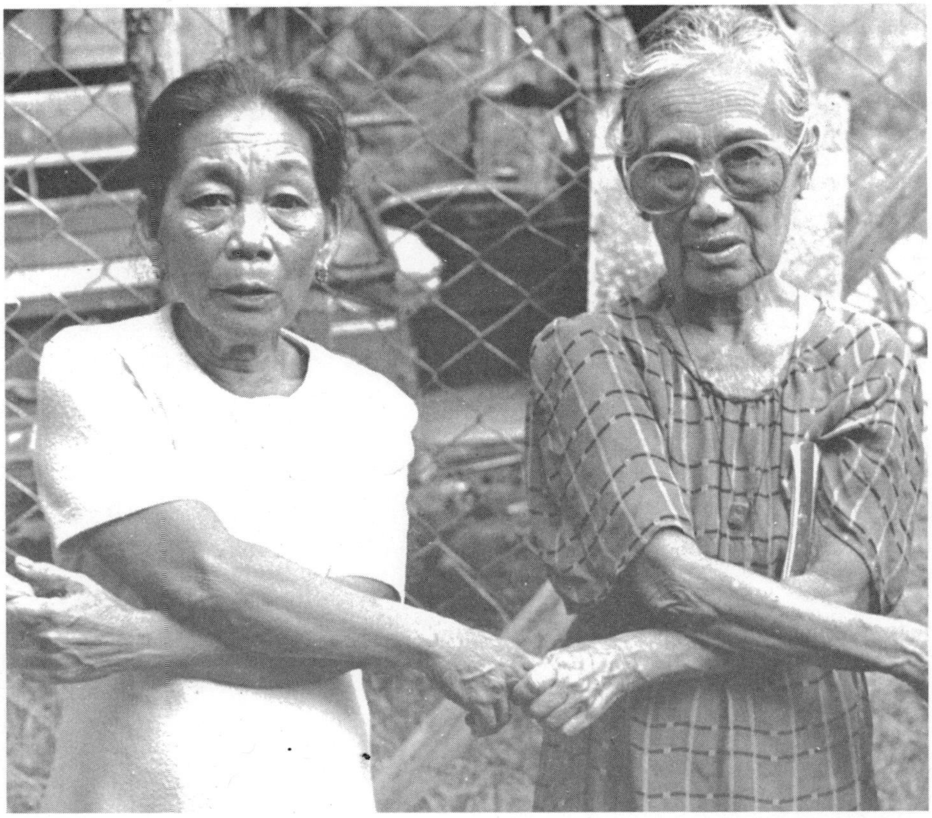

Photo courtesy of Coalition of Services for the Elderly, Inc. (COSE)

Groups provide support and understanding.

The **goals** for most groups are to:

- share experiences so that people recognize they are not alone in their experiences;
- gain support and understanding from one another;
- help resocialize older persons and improve feelings of belonging;
- exchange information and learn techniques which promote positive mental health; and
- increase independence, self-care and mental stimulation for those who have regressed and those who have memory deficits.

Remotivation therapy

In this group work, the focus is on simple (routine) activities of day-to-day living which make one feel *productive*. The interaction usually does not explore feelings in depth. Instead, the group leader helps the older persons to (a) think about activities which were done in the past, (b) consider how and why the activities gave them feelings of productivity, (c) compare the past to their present situation, and (d) explore current and reasonable activities which can provide motivation and accomplishment. The group is usually held several times a week for a few months. At the end of that time, the group may no longer be needed.

Reminiscence Groups

Reminiscence has been described as part of a normal life review process which occurs in all people, brought about by an awareness of one's closeness to death in later years. It is characterized by (a) a review of past experiences, (b) dealing with unresolved conflicts, feelings of guilt or failure, (c) recalling one's successes, (d) in order to achieve personal integration of events in one's life in the final years, and (e) to gain peace and serenity. *The review of one's life in this way is considered to contribute to psychologically healthy aging.*

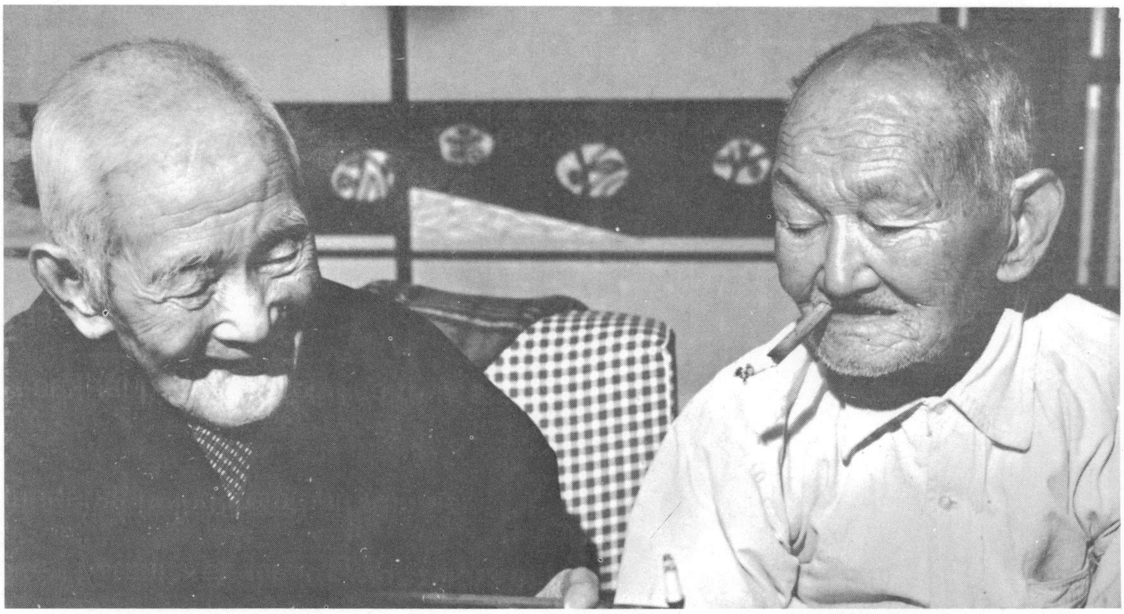

Photo courtesy of Tokyo Metropolitan Institute of Gerontology

The continuance of relatively high levels of intellectual activity are essential to the maintenance of brain function in old age, so it is important that friendships and activities with significant others are promoted.

Elderly are guided (a) to recall persons and events (both happy and sad, disappointing and hopeful and so on) in their lives which have given meaning and purpose in life, (b) to explore happenings about which they have regret, (c) to identify ways of resolving things about which they have regret, (d) to reconcile discrepancies between what actually happened in life and the hopes of what was to be, and (e) to consider the totality of one's life experience.

The *sharing of memories* can cover any *stage of life*, many subjects such as *holidays*, *major life events*, *relationships* with families, friends and co-workers, and *accomplishments*. The group averages in size from six to eight older persons, and meetings are held once or twice a week for about one hour. The number of weeks that the group continues varies. Use of family albums, scrapbooks, genealogies and other memorabilia can help to develop the topics.

According to recent work by Watt and Wong (1991), there are actually six types of reminiscence: integrative, instrumental, transmissive, narrative, escapist, and obsessive.

Integrative - *This is the classic model of reminiscence* in which older persons review their life in preparation for death in order to achieve peace and continuity with the past.

Instrumental - This type of reminiscence involves reviewing challenging situations which happened in the past, and the strategies which were used successfully to overcome the experience, *in order to problem-solve* some current difficulty. A particular *goal* in this type of reminiscence is to give the aged person a sense of personal control over a present difficulty.

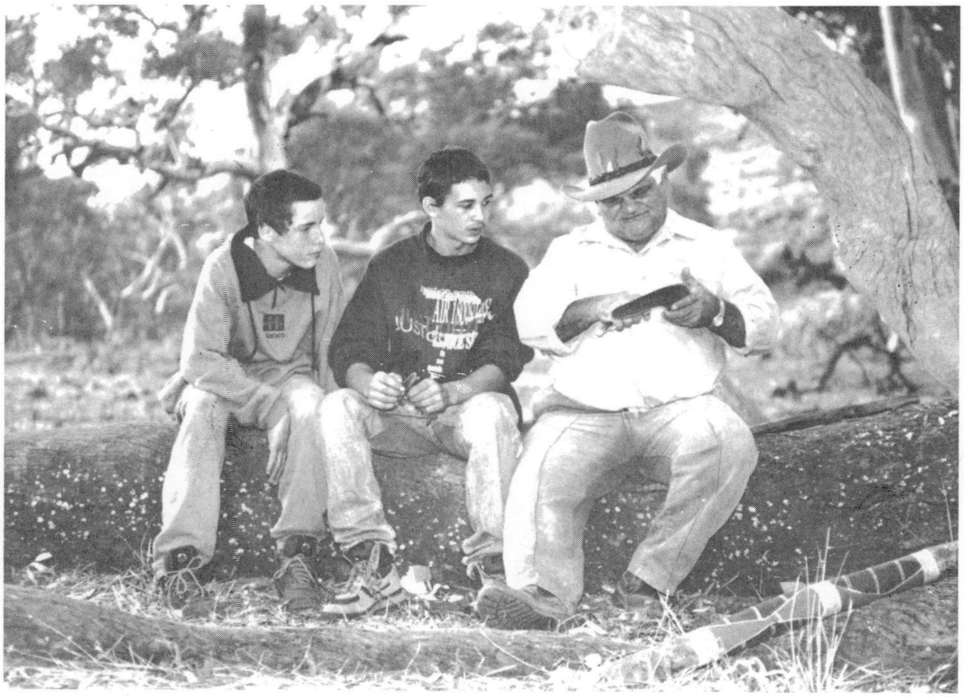

Photo courtesy of Narelle Autio

Learning about making a boomerang from Aboriginal elderly involves pleasant communication.

Transmissive - In reminiscing this way, *the person passes on to a younger generation*, thoughts of *wisdom* which s/he has gained over the many years. Most older people have a need to contribute to society in this way, and to relate life experiences which help support the why and how of *value systems*. Often the examples told include lessons discovered in experiences of war (such as honour), marriage (such as love), child-rearing (such as patience), and so forth.

Narrative - This is *a form of storytelling*. It is usually limited to describing memories of the past simply to provide facts about one's personal story in life. Pleasure is gained in recalling past times which are remembered with fondness or satisfaction.

Escapist - This is a form of *denial*. The person focuses only on the positive or happy events of the past as a way of ignoring an unhappy present. Although *it can have some positive effects* by reducing the pain or sadness of a bad situation (such as being in a nursing home, or being disabled and homebound), it can *cause one to disengage*, thereby *reducing* the older person's ability to *cope* with current demands.

Obsessive - With this type of life review, the older person thinks of nothing but the negative and upsetting events of the past and has strong feelings of guilt, despair, shame and the like. This is *not* conducive to healthy aging and needs specific professional treatment by referral to a mental health specialist.

(Watt & Wong, 1991)

There are several other types of groups which help to sustain the elderly and their families.

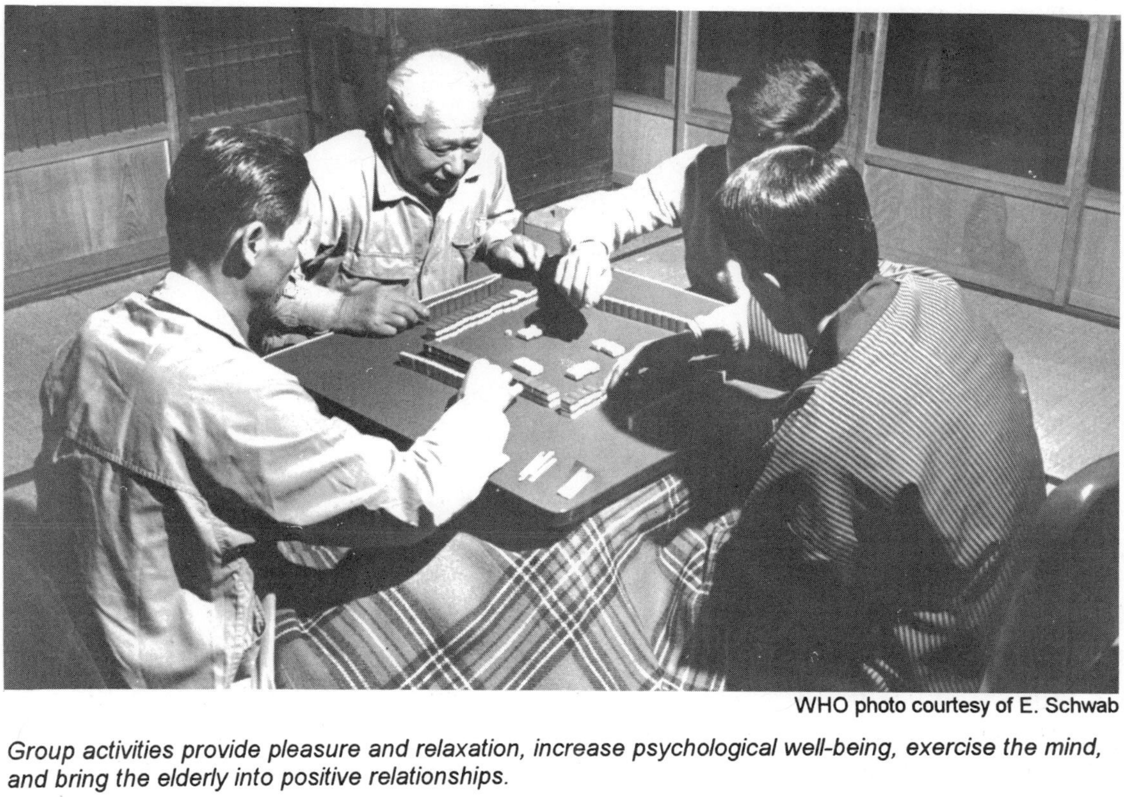

WHO photo courtesy of E. Schwab

Group activities provide pleasure and relaxation, increase psychological well-being, exercise the mind, and bring the elderly into positive relationships.

Music groups, art therapy groups and poetry groups

All these groups have similar goals which are to (a) provide pleasure and relaxation, (b) increase psychological well-being, (c) stimulate movement and exercise of the body and mind, and (d) bring persons who are withdrawn into relating better with others. The size and timing of the group can vary easily depending upon the resources available.

Music groups use music to express feelings. In village communities, the elderly are an important part of music festivals. Some include singing or sing-along, others provide members with musical instruments to play, and sometimes even dancing or other forms of movement are included. Although in urban centres, these groups are usually led by someone talented in music, records, tapes and radios can also be used by anyone who desires to start a group. The type of instruments, dance and music depends on the talent available from members and leaders. This type of group can accommodate a large number of elderly people.

Art therapy and poetry groups gather older people together to create and enjoy various forms of artistry. Almost any medium and project can be done such as making Origami birds out of construction paper, making decorations from yarn, drawing pictures, using fabric to quilt, weaving baskets, reading many different kinds of poetry and so on.

Groups for the elderly who are grieving over death of loved ones

As people age, they experience the death of increasing numbers of friends and relatives. These may include the death of neighbors, spouses and children. The goals of the groupwork are (a) to assist older persons to adjust to the loss of the loved one, (b) to support the person in the most difficult first months following the event(s), and (c) to prevent later problems from unresolved grief. The discussion centres around *expressing sadness* and *talking about the importance of the relationship* and the *wonderful memories*. It is suggested that persons trained in the mental health speciality be employed to conduct such groups.

Groups for family members

These groups can be formed for many *purposes* such as (1) to *educate* families about the aging process or the illness of the older person, (2) to gain family *cooperation* in the plan of care for the elderly, and (3) to *reduce anxiety, guilt, frustration* and/or *burden* about the elderly to whom they are providing care.

Group work centres on (a) identifying the problems or issues, (b) providing information, (c) exploring how the family has managed problems in the past, (d) helping family members to build on their strengths in past problem solving experiences, and (e) assisting them to get needed resources of support. Again, these groups are best conducted by health care workers who have expertise in the mental health sciences when available, as opposed to health care workers who are generalists.

NOTE: **Module 11 (Supporting families in caregiving) contains additional information about helping families.**

Depression

The most common mental health problem in older persons is ***depression***. *Chronic illness, pain, death of loved ones*, frustration with *limitations* in activities of daily living **(ADLs)**, or *lack of control* over one's life and activities may all contribute. Depression robs one of the enjoyment of living and interferes with quality of life. Associated with depression in the elderly is the possibility of suicide, especially in men.

In older people, depression may appear very similar to confusion and dementia. The symptoms can be so closely related that term ***pseudodementia*** is sometimes used. Many of the *symptoms* of depression are the same as those of dementia. For example *difficulty concentrating* and *poor memory.*

Depression is characterized by feelings of sadness, pessimism, and hopelessness. Symptoms may include:

1. statements such as "I don't have any reason to go on living", "I don't have any energy";
2. behaviour such as crying;
3. excessive or frequent drinking of alcohol;
4. loss of interest or pleasure in most activities;
5. unkempt appearance;
6. lack of appetite;
7. refusing to take medications which have been prescribed;
8. sleeping more than usual;
9. complaining of many health problem; and
10. paranoid feelings.

In older persons there is sometimes ***agitated depression*** which means that there is:

1. excessive physical activity;
2. pacing;
3. failure to sleep;
4. constant appetite and eating;
5. irritability; and
6. hostility.

Assessment of depression includes making observations of the older person's behaviour, and asking questions of both the elderly and the family concerning the older person's mood. Use of a standardized depression assessment instrument can be helpful in suspected depression. One such instrument is the **Geriatric Depression Scale** (**GDS**) (Sheikh & Yesavage, 1986**)**. *This instrument was developed specifically for use with the elderly,* employs a yes/no format and is simple and quick to administer. The higher the total score, the greater the indication of depression.

(Both the long and short versions of the Geriatric Depression Scale can be found on pages 13-14).

Screening may be done with either the original 30-item form (Yesavage, et al., 1983) or with the 15-item short version. Although the tool is recommended for assessing depressive symptomatology typical of older persons, it should be employed with three cautions.

First, *it is not intended to diagnose depression*, but only to serve as *an adjunct to case-finding*. Second, *it is most accurate in cognitively intact older persons and in the 30-item version* (Brink, et al., 1991; Burke, et al., 1989). Third, *the short form (15 items) is more susceptible than the long form to ethnic and cultural variations* (Cwikel & Ritchie, 1988; 1989).

Somatic complaints must be thoroughly evaluated to be certain that there is no physical basis for the depression. Severe depression may require electroconvulsive therapy **(ECT)** (Butler & Lewis, 1977) *or* antidepressant medications may be prescribed. Individual or group therapy will likely be recommended, and this source of support is important for the family caregivers as well as for the depressed elderly.

There is evidence that *loss of control* has a negative effect on people (regardless of age) including (1) contributing to depression, (2) developing disease, and (3) slowing recovery. For older people there may be many sources for loss of control for example due to retirement, lack of money or need for assistance.

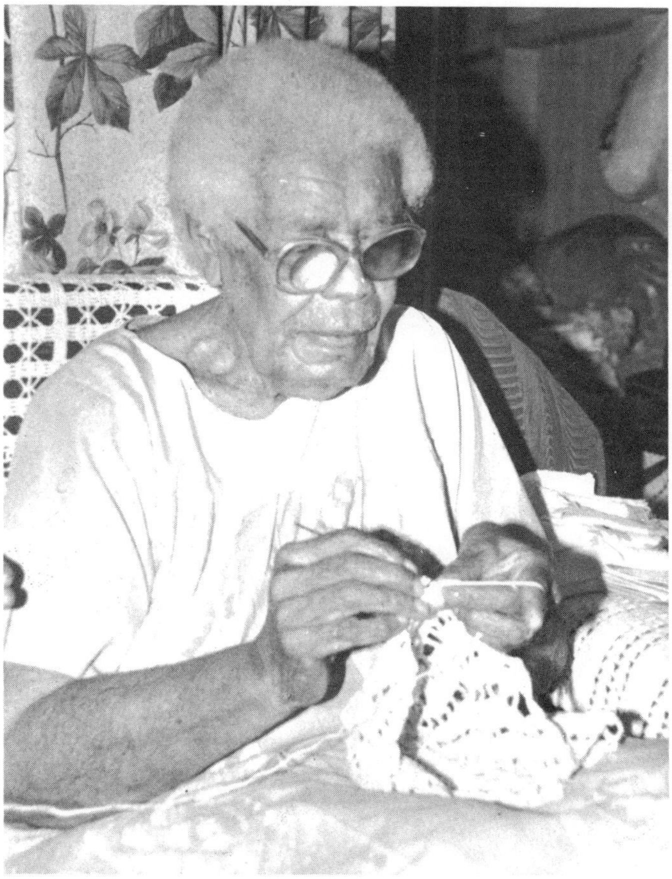

Photo courtesy of T. Miller

This 87-year old Fijian nurse says, "I like to live alone, so I can read my bible. I cherish my independence." However, she enjoys frequent visits from villagers who live in the same community.

Try to find some areas where the older person can have control, such as:

1. decision-making about the schedule of daily activities;
2. what foods to plan for meals;
3. what products to buy for family grocery shopping; and
4. how to handle a particular situation with the grandchildren.

Physical decline associated with aging can be reduced by changing the environment to enhance control.

Engaging the person in *physical activity* has been found to *reduce stress*. Aerobic exercise, walking, swimming and Tai Chi are all excellent forms of stress-reducing exercise.

Exercise A

As a group, discuss the cultural influences in your country(ies) which may prevent older persons and their families from admitting that they need help in the form of mental health services. Suggest ways that these barriers can be overcome.

Exercise B

Imagine yourself at 80 years of age. Write down what you expect to be happening in your life. Then have students divide into pairs and administer the Geriatric Depression Scale to one another. Have students share with the group, how they pictured themselves in their situations at 80 years of age and how they scored on the depression scale.

Short-answer exercise

1. What is the purpose of reminiscence?

2. How do you think you could determine whether agitation in an older person was due to depression?

Bibliography

Anders, R.L. & Kanai-Pak, M. (1988). Growing old in Japan. World Health, (December): 8-11.

Bergmann, K.(1978). Neurosis and personality disorder in old age. In A.D. Isaacs & F. Post (Eds). Studies in geriatric psychiatry. (pp. 41-76) New York: Wiley.

Boxwell, A.O. (1988). Geriatric suicide: The preventable death. Nurse Practitioner, 13(6): 10, 11, 15, 18, 19.

Brink, T.L., Yesavage, J.A., Owen, L., Heersema, P.H., Adey,M., & Rose, T.L. (1982). Screening tests for geriatric depression. Clinical Gerontology, 3: 57-59.

Buckwater, K.C. (1990). How to unmask depression. Geriatric Nursing. 11(4): 179-181.

Burnside, I.M. (Ed.)(1978). Working with the elderly: Group processes and techniques. North Scituate, MA: Duxbury Press.

Burnside, I. (1992). Reminiscence and life review: Analysing each concept. Journal of Advanced Nursing, 17: 855-862.

Butler, R.N. & Lewis, M.I. (1982) (3rd ed.). Aging and mental health : Positive psychosocial and biomedical approaches. St. Louis: C.V. Mosby.

Butler, R.N. (1992). Aging and mental health - diagnosis of dementia and depression. Geriatrics, 47(6): 49-52, 55-57.

Cadoret, R.J. & Widmer, R.B. (1988). The development of depressive symptoms in elderly following onset of severe physical illness. Journal of Family Practice, 27(1): 71-76.

Carucci, G. et al. (1988). Trazodone in late life depressive states: A double-blind multicenter study. Psychopharmacology, 95 Supplement: S34-S36.

Dana, R.H. (Ed.)(1981). Human services for cultural minorities. Baltimore: University Park Press.

Emery, G. (1981). Cognitive therapy with the elderly. In G. Emery, S.D. Hollon & R.C. Bedrosian (Eds.). New directions in cognitve therapy, New York: Guilford.

Frank-Stromborg, M. & Olsen, S.J. (1993). Cancer prevention in minority populations: Cultural implications for health care professionals. St. Louis: Mosby.

Gallagher, D. & Thompson, L.W. (1983). Effectiveness of psychotherapy for both endogenous and non-endogenous depression in older adult out-patients. Journal of Gerontology, 38: 707-712.

Garrett, J.E. (1987). Multiple losses in older adults. Journal of Gerontological Nursing, 13:8-12.

Haggerty, J.J., Golden, R.N., Evans, D.L. & Janowsky, D.S. (1988). Differential diagnosis of pseudodementia in the elderly. Geriatrics, 43(3): 61-69, 72, 74.

Herr, K.A. (1992). Geriatric mental health - Chronic pain and depression. Journal of Psychosocial Nursing and Mental Health Services, 30(9): 7-12, 38-39.

Kane, R.A. & Kane, R.L. (1981). Assessing the elderly: A practical guide to measurement. Lexington,MA: D.C. Heath & Company.

Keane, S.M. & Sells, S. (1990). Recognizing depression in the elderly. Journal of Gerontological Nursing, 16(1): 21-25.

Kimmel, D.C. (1990). Adulthood and aging: An interdisciplinary, developmental view (3rd ed.).New York: John Wiley & Sons.

Lewinsohn, P.M. (1975). The behavioural study and treatment of depression. In M. Hersen, R. Eisler & P. Miller (Eds.). Progress in behavior modification vol.1, London: Academic Press.

Lewis, M.I. & Butler, R.N.(1974). Life review therapy: Putting memories to work in individual and group psychotherapy. Geriatrics, 29: 165-174.

Matteson, M.A. & McConnell, E.S. (1988). Gerontological nursing: Concepts and practice. Philadelphia: W.B. Saunders.

Nelson, P.B. (1989). Ethnic differences in intrinsic/extrinsic religious orientation and depression in the elderly. Archives of Psychiatric Nursing, 3(4): 199-204.

Reed, P.G. (1989). Mental health of older adults. Western Journal of Nursing Research, 11(12): 143-157.

Rockwell, E., Lam, R.W. & Zisook, S. (1988). Antidepressant drug studies in the elderly. Psychiatric Clinics of North America, 11(1): 215-233.

Rodin, J., Mc Avay, G. & Timko, C. (1988). A longitudinal study of depressed mood and sleep disturbances in elderly. Journal of Gerontology, 43(2): P45-P53.

Sarafino, E.P. (1990). Health psychology: Biopsychosocial interactions. New York: John Wiley & Sons.

Seligman, M. (1975). Helplessness: On depression, development and death. San Francisco: W.H. Freeman.

Sheikh, J.I. & Yesavage, J.A. (1986). Geriatric depression scale (GDS) recent evidence and development of a shorter version. Clinical Gerontologist, 5: 165-172.

Sorenson, S.B. (1991). Suicide among the elderly: Issues facing public health. American Journal of Public Health, 81(9): 1109-1110.

Sparacino, J.(1978-9). Individual psychotherapy with the aged: A selective review. International Journal of Ageing & Human Development, 9(3): 197-217.

Steiner, D., & Marcopulous, B. (1991). Depression in the elderly: Characteristics and clinical management. Nursing Clinics of North America, 26(3): 585-600.

Sweer, L., Martin, D.C., Ladd, R.A., Miller, J.K. & Karpf, M. (1988). The medical evaluation of elderly patients with major depression. Journal of Gerontology, 43(3): M53-M58.

Watt, L.M. & Wong, P.T.P. (1991). A taxonomy of reminiscence and therapeutic implications. Journal of Gerontological Social Work, 16(1/2): 37-57.

Williams, A.K. & Schulz, R. (1988). Association of pain and physical dependency with depression in physically ill middle-aged and elderly persons. Physical Therapy, 68(8): 1226-1230.

Wolanin, M.O. & Phillips, L.R.F. (1981). Confusion: Prevention and care. St. Louis: C.V. Mosby.

Wood, K.A., Harris, M.J., Morreale, A. & Rizos, A.L. (1988). Drug induced psychosis and depression in the elderly. Psychiatric Clinics of North America, 11(1): 167-193.

Woods, R.Y. & Britton, P.G. (1985). Clinical psychology with the elderly. Rockville,MD.:Aspen Systems.

Yesavage, J., Brink, T., Rose, T., Lum, O., Adey, V. & Leirer, V. (1983). Development and validation of a geriatric depression screening scale: A preliminary report. Journal of Psychiatric Research, 17: 37-49.

Zorumski, C.F., Rubin, E.H. & Burke, W.J. (1988). Electroconvulsive therapy for the elderly: A review. Hospital & Community Psychiatry, 39(6): 643-647.

Caregiving

MODULE 11 - *SUPPORTING FAMILIES IN CAREGIVING*

Objectives

On completion of this module, the student should be able to:

1. explain the concept of "caregiver burden";
2. describe risks to older persons and families that result from sustained and unrelieved caregiver burden;
3. recognize mistreatment of an older person; and
4. develop care plans (with goals and interventions) for caregiver support and ways of evaluating the effectiveness.

Supporting families in caregiving

Families provide the majority of care to their older relatives. Although this practice is not new, changes in society have made the care more complicated. All people are living longer and this has increased the number of generations living together, sometimes up to as many as three to five generations. In countries where housing is very expensive and living space is small, it can be hard to accomodate both the elderly parents and other family members. This is especially true if the older person uses a walker or a wheelchair. It can pose problems by limiting the personal space and *privacy* of all family members.

Traditionally, women have been responsible for the care of the elderly, including daughters and daughters-in-law. In many countries there is a trend for increasing numbers of women to be employed outside the home. This may result in the eldest child (a son or a daughter who may be in his or her 70s) having to care for parents (who may be in their 80s or 90s). It can be much more demanding for older people to care for the "old-old" than might be expected for younger persons.

If the older person is frail or impaired, family caregivers experience what is called **caregiver burden**. These are the physical, emotional, social, and financial costs associated with the caregiving experience. The caregiver has been referred to as the "hidden patient" because most of the attention of health care workers is directed towards meeting the needs of the patient, rather than the caregiver.

The caregiver is as much in need of care and attention as the older person.

If the needs of the caregiver are ignored over time, the well-being of the caregiver may decline, a change in living situation may result for the older person, and the quality of life of the entire family may be affected negatively.

The **goals** of supporting the caregiver and relieving burden are to:

- maintain the physical and mental health of the caregiver;
- gain cooperation on goals to be achieved in caring for the older person;
- avoid development of an abusive situation;
- reduce the risk of institutionalization for the older person; and
- promote quality of life for the entire family.

The physical and mental health of the caregiver

The physical and emotional health of the caregiver can be threatened by **stress** which occurs in the course of trying to give needed care to the older person, while at the same time trying to meet ongoing responsibilities of work and caring for other family members.

Assessing the extent of burden is difficult because caregiver burden is both an objective and subjective experience.

Objective factors are those which can be observed and include such things as (1) the *age* and *physical health* of the caregiver, (2) the *amount of care* the older person requires, (3) the number and nature of *additional responsibilities* brought about by the cargiving, (4) the *length of time the care has been required* and *how long it is expected to continue*, (5) the *time spent in caregiving* compared to *opportunities for free time* or *time away from* the caregiving situation, (6) the number and type of *support systems available* to the caregiver, and (7) the *added financial costs* which may come about in caring for the older person.

Subjective factors are those burdens which concern the psychological and emotional response of the caregiver such as (1) feelings of *fatigue*, (2) feeling *conflict* between what one should or must do for the elder and what one (or needs) wants to do, (3) feeling *resentful*, and (4) feeling *overwhelmed*.

Some of the negative feelings of caregiving may be balanced in part by the positive feelings of being useful. However, in an attempt to be helpful, caregivers can actually make the older person more dependent. This is called **Induced dependency** (Kuypers & Bengston, 1984; Avorn & Langer, 1982). Helping with self-care (such as dressing and feeding) beyond that required has been found to reduce the older persons' ability to perform care activities themselves. The elderly learns to rely on the caregiver for things he or she is capable of doing, *thereby causing even more work and burden for the caregiver*. Sometimes caregivers create this situation unintentionally because it is often easier and/or faster to do things for the elderly than to let him or her do things for him/herself.

Here are some examples of how caregivers make older persons more dependent (that is, induce dependency). Typically, frail elderly eat very slowly, and getting them to finish a meal takes a great deal of time. There is evidence that when older people are slow to feed themselves *they are often fed because it is faster*. Another example is that although most old people can walk, they walk very slowly. Caregivers may let them sit for long periods or let them use wheelchairs, when walking them would be better for their strength and mobility.

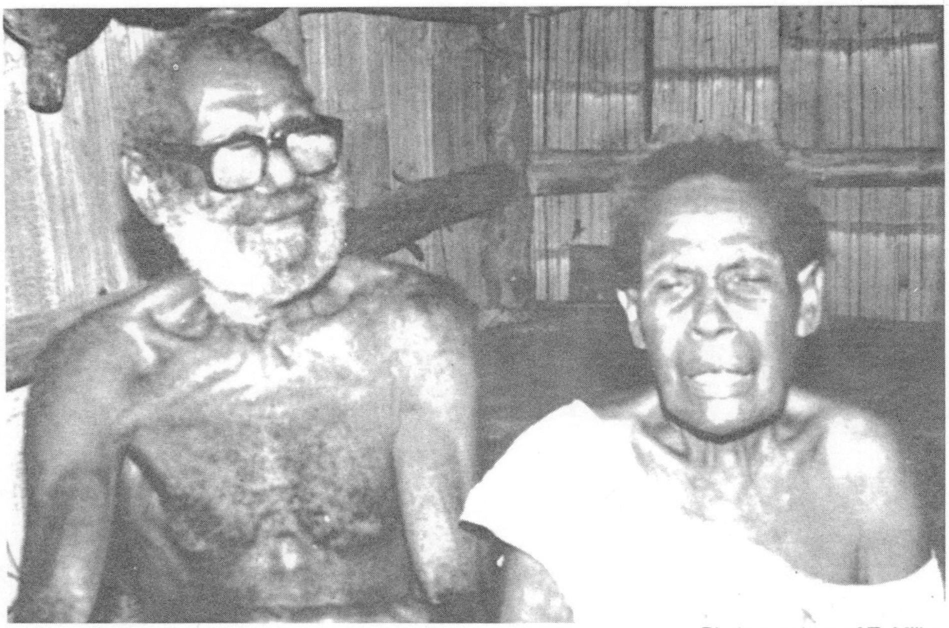

Photo courtesy of T. Miller

"At 80 plus, I find taking care of my husband who is almost blind to be very difficult. I am in constant pain from the work", says Vanuatu village grandmother. Thus, it is important to be aware of the emotional and physical needs of this village wife who is the caregiver.

Caregivers often do not admit that they need help and resist seeking and/or accepting help for cultural or religious reasons. They may believe that (1) emotional pain should be endured because suffering is repayment for bad deeds, (2) the situation is entirely in God's hands, or (3) they want to appear strong to maintain their dignity, to people outside of the family. However, if the emotional needs of the caregiver are not given attention, the stress builds and caregivers are pushed beyond their limits. This then can lead to problems in the entire family, decline of the physical health of the caregiver, and the chance that the elderly is ABUSED or is sent away to an institution.

It is not uncommon for emotional stress to be disguised as complaints of headache, backache, neckache, stomach problems, and sleeping difficulties.

Abuse of the elderly

This can be of one of two types, mistreatment or neglect.

Mistreatment includes *physical mistreatment* such as tying the person in chair or in bed for long periods of time, handling the person roughly, and striking the person, and *psychological mistreatment* such as shouting or threatening the person, and treating the elderly as if he or she is as a child.

Neglect can also be of a physical or psychological nature. *Physical neglect* means failing to provide something which is needed. Examples are (1) not giving medications properly and on time, (2) not providing adequate fluid or nutrition, (3) allowing an unsafe living environment, (4) not making arrangements for the hygiene and elimination needs of the older person, and (5) being unreasonably slow to attend to the elderly's medical and health care needs. *Psychological neglect* includes isolating or ignoring the elderly, and depriving them of their rights and choices. An example of ignoring an elderly is leaving the person to sit alone for long periods without conversation or activities to occupy him or her.

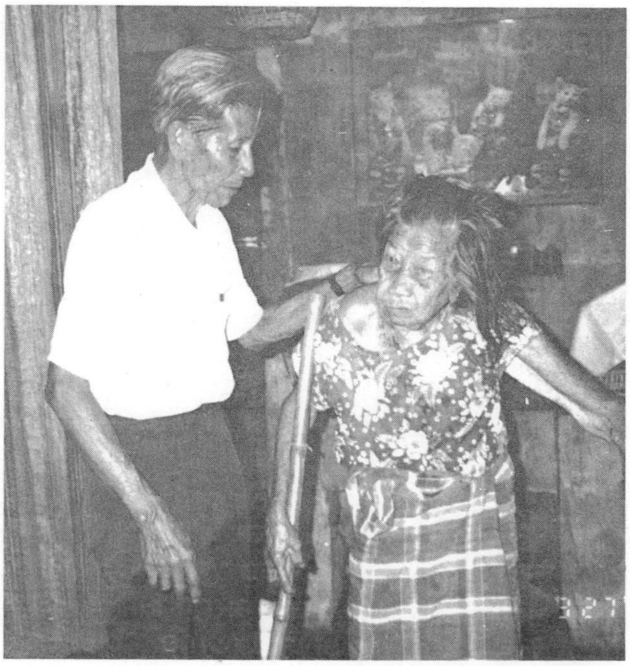

Photo courtesy of L.A. Baldago

It is essential to provide support to caregivers of the elderly at home, in order that they can provide adequate care. In Iloilo (Philippines), this 70-year old lady is being taken cared of by her 64-year old brother.

Usually when abusive situations arise, it is not an *isolated event*, and *more than one type of abuse is occurring*. Elderly abuse is a very sensitive issue and often very difficult to detect. Here are some warning signs.

Signs or *indications* of mistreatment or neglect might include:

- there are skin injuries such as cuts, skin tears or bruises or untreated bedsores (pressure sores);
- the explanation offered by the family for the skin injuries does not seem to make sense (that is, it does not seem probable or reasonable);
- there is a pattern to the cuts and bruises (for example, they appear on both arms, or only on the face);

- there are signs of malnutrition or dehydration and the caregiver is very vague and unclear about the diet, fluid intake and so on;
- the older person is repeatedly found to be soiled by urine or faeces and/or is not very clean overall;
- the older person is left alone a lot and seems not to have much to do for enjoyment;
- the older person seems afraid to talk or interact with you, especially when asked questions about how things are going in his or her life or when asked about cuts and bruises;
- the older person is in need of medical attention but the caregiver has not obtained the necessary care; and
- medications and other instructions for care of the older person are not followed despite teaching and review of how and what to do.

IMPLICATIONS AND RECOMMENDATIONS

Family caregivers need a high level of knowledge and skills, and much emotional support. Assessment should begin with finding out exactly (1) what care must be provided for the elderly (such as feeding, dressing, bathing and toileting), (2) what the older person is capable of doing for him or herself, (3) how much extra time is spent by the caregiver in preparing meals, houskeeping, and laundry, (4) what arrangements exist to give the caregiver rest and relaxation, and (5) what resources and support systems are available to the caregiver.

Physical health complaints by a caregiver should make one suspect that they need more assistance in the home. Maintaining *awareness of cultural and religious influences*, and *establishing trust* with the caregiver are essential to making it acceptable for him or her to accept help.

For example, a caregiver may avoid seeking relief from symptoms of emotional stress (headache, stomach irritation) at the beginning of a new year, if it is believed that this will incline one to be ill all year. Trust is built by:

- keeping lines of communication open;
- requesting suggestions from the caregiver and other family members;
- avoiding judgements about the home situation;
- showing support by listening to concerns; and

- involving the caregiver and family in decisions about the care of the elderly relative.

In some cultures, respect for authority and the value of harmony may make the caregiver feel it is not acceptable to express disagreement to suggestions offered. The more one can build trust, the more likely the caregiver will feel comfortable in expressing a difference in opinion, and hence, the more likely it will be that the plan for correction will be realistic and acted upon.

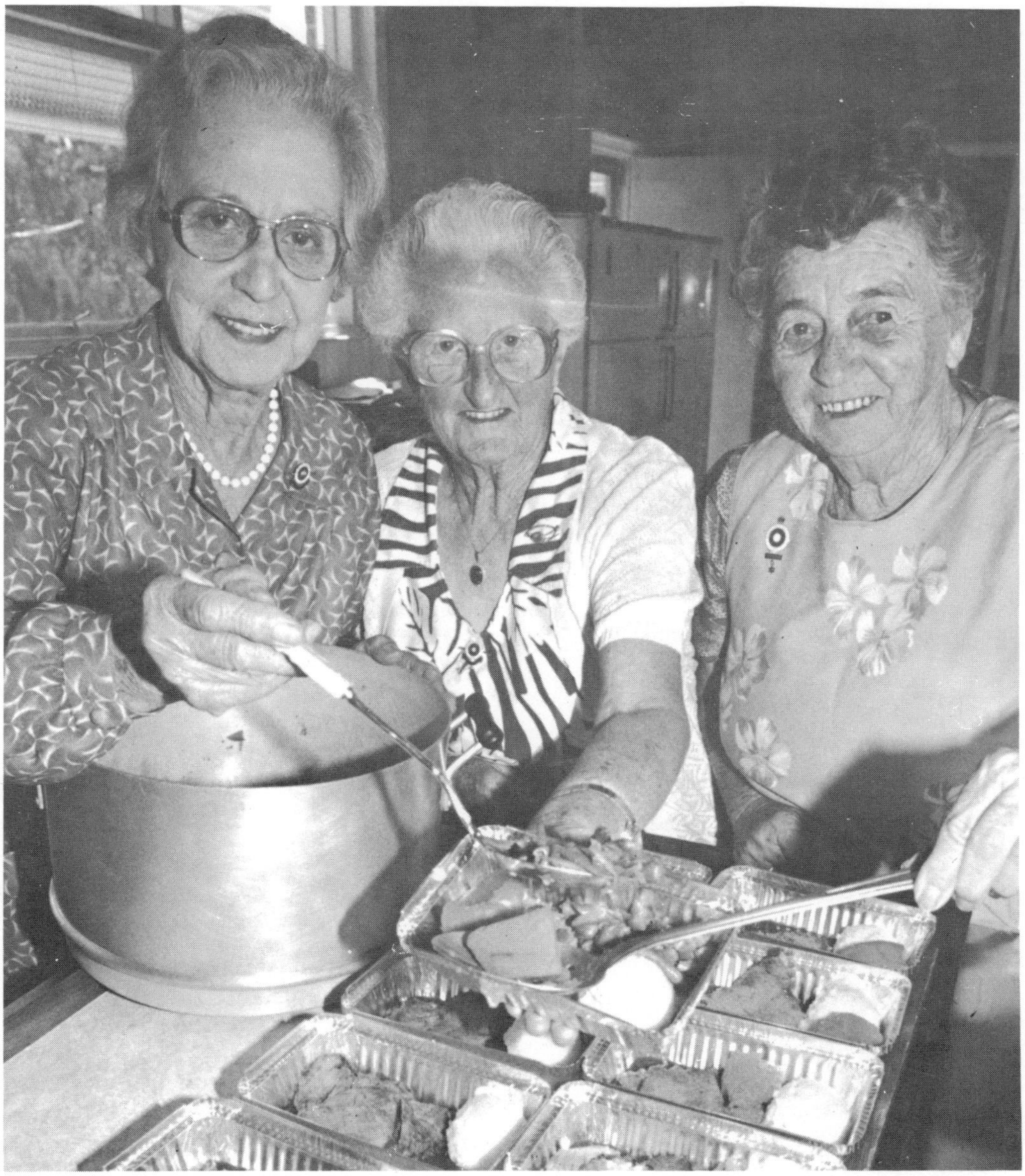

Photo courtesy of The Advertiser

"Meals on Wheels" support the eldely's ability to live at home. There are 9000 Meals on Wheels volunteers in South Australia who provide meals for those who are unable to cook for themselves.

Identify ways in which the older person can be made more independent. Assess the functional capacity of the older person in relationship to barriers in the home environment. Most limitations centre around toileting, meal preparation, and dressing. Analyse how the design of things can be modified and what adaptive equipment or appliances might be useful.

Search for ways of *motivating the elderly* as much as possible. Motivation may depend upon cultural factors. For example, recently it was found that for Japanese elderly, those who had *social participation* in organized activity lived longer than those who simply had social contact in terms of visiting (Sugisawa, Liang & Liu, 1994). Examples of activities that the elderly can become involved in include (1) working as an adviser or honourary official, (2) participating in voluntary associations of retired persons, (3) helping with neighbourhood work teams, (4) attending workshops, (5) attending clinics where cultural and recreational opportunities are offered, such as films and artistic performances, (6) participating in educational programmes about nutrition, hygiene, and disease prevention such as are offered in Korea, and (7) visiting historical places and recreation centres.

Based on the policies which governments have in place, countries differ in what social support systems, both formal and informal *and* in home and community, are available. Most caregivers do not know how to go about getting or using support services. Therefore, *coordination* of the network between public community health services plus private sector resources is a major role for health care workers in helping caregivers.

Examples of services include:

- Ministries of Health and Social Affairs;
- Community health practitioners for rural areas;
- Geriatric Specialty Services which provide house calls;
- Day hospitals,
- Outpatient services, inpatient care for investigation of major problems;
- Day-care centres, senior centres which provide activities and nutritious meals;
- Council of housing programmes to improve housing arrangements and living environments; and
- Respite care, which is aimed at sharing the burden of care with family and other informal caregivers.

Exercise A

You have been advised that an older person in the community is being abused. The family has been struggling to care for the older person for several years now. The older person has a dementing illness, probably Alzheimer's disease, and is now incontinent of both urine and faeces.

Role-play the situation. How can you further assess whether abuse is taking place? What can be done to help this older person and the family?

Exercise B

Develop a care plan (with goals and interventions) for caregiver support and ways of evaluating the effectiveness. The plan may relate to the situation described in exercise A or some other one of your choice or the instructor's choice.

Short-answer exercise

1. List the resources in your area of your country which could be used to help support caregivers. Include public and private, and formal and informal.

2. Describe what resources are absent from your community and what can be done to compensate for the absence of these services. Are there more deficiencies in the public or private sector, the formal or informal network?

Bibliography

Anders, R.L. & Kanai-Pak, M. (1988). Growing old in Japan. World Health, (December): 8-11.

Avorn, J., & Langer, E. (1982). Induced disability in nursing home patients: A controlled trial. Journal of the American Geriatrics Society, 30(6): 397-400.

Baltes, M. M., Honn, S., Barton, E. M., Orzech, M., & Lago, D. (1983). On the social ecology of dependence and independence in elderly nursing home residents. Journal of Gerontology, 38(5): 556-564.

Breckman, R.S. & Adelman, R.D. (1988). Strategies for helping victims of elder mistreatment. Newbury Park, CA: Sage Publications.

Czaja, S.J., Weber, R.A. & Nair, S.N. (1993). A human factors analysis of ADL activities: A capability-demand approach. The Journals of Gerontology, 4(Special Issue): 44-48.

Fagin, C.M. (1990). Nursing leadership: Global strategies. New York: National League for Nursing.

Frank-Stromborg, M. & Olsen, S.J. (1993). Cancer prevention in minority populations: Cultural implications for health care professionals. St. Louis: Mosby.

Godlove, C., Dunn, G., & Wright, H. (1980). Caring for old people in New York and London: The nurses' aid interviews. Journal of the Royal Society of Medicine, 73(10): 713-723.

Gudykunst, W.B. (1991). Bridging differences: Effective intergroup communication. Newbury Park, CA: Sage Publications.

Kavanagh, K.H. & Kennedy, P.H. (1992). Promoting cultural diversity: Strategies for health care professionals. Newbury Park, CA: Sage Publications.

Kimmel, D.C. (1990). Adulthood and aging: An interdisciplinary, developmental view (3rd ed.).New York: John Wiley & Sons.

Kuypers, J. A., & Bengston, V. L. (1984). Perspectives on the older family. In W.H. Quinn, & G.A. Hughston (Eds.), Independent aging: Family and social systems perspectives, (pp. 2-20). Rockville, MD: Aspen Publishers.

Langer, E. J. (1979). The illusion of incompetence. In L. Perlmutter, & R. Monty (Eds.). Choice and perceived control, (pp. 301-313). New York: Lawrence Erlbaum Associates.

Langer, E. J., & Benevento, A. (1978). Self-induced dependence. Journal of personality and social psychology, 36(8): 886-893.

Lipman, A., Slater, R., & Harris, H. (1979). The quality of verbal interaction in homes for old people. Gerontology, 25(5): 275-284.

Pawlson, G., Goodwin, M., & Keith, K. (1986). Wheelchair use by ambulatory nursing home residents. Journal of the American Geriatrics Society, 34(12): 860-864.

Pruchno, R.A., Kleban, M.H., Michaels, J.E. & Dempsey, N.P. (1990). Mental and physical health of caregiving spouses: Development of a causal model. Journal of Gerontology, 45(5): P192-199.

Rogers, J. C., & Snow, T. (1982). An assessment of the feeding behaviours of the institutionalized elderly. American Journal of Occupational Therapy, 36(6): 375-380.

Schulz, R., Visintainer, P. & Williamson, G.M. (1990). Psychiatric and physical morbidity effects of caregiving. Journal of Gerontology, 45(5): P181-P191.

Seligman, M. (1975). On depression, development and death. San Francisco: W.H. Freeman.

Sharlin, S. A., & Polansky, N. A. (1972). The process of infantilization. American Journal of Orthopsychiatry, 42(1): 92- 102.

Stanford, E.P. & Torres-Gil, F.M. (Eds.)(1992). Diversity: New approaches to ethnic aging. Amityville, NY: Baywood Publishing Company Inc.

Sugisawa, H., Liang, J. & Liu, X. (19940. Social networks, social support, and mortality among older people in Japan. Journal of Gerontology, 49(1): S3-S13.

The Arizona Long Term Care Gerontology Center (September 1990). Alzheimer's disease: Pieces of the puzzle. University of Arizona, Tucson, AZ.

Van Ort, S., & Phillips, L. R. (1992). Observations of feeding behaviours in nursing home residents. Geriatric Nursing, 249-253.

Health Promotion Summary

MODULE 12 - *HEALTH PROMOTION SUMMARY*

Objectives

On completion of this module, the student should be able to:

1. describe needs for health promotion in the elderly, including sleep and exercise, nutrition, screening, case-finding and referral, prevention of smoking and alcohol abuse, accident prevention and medication management;

2. Enumerate strategies for health promotion in regard to the needs; and

3. Develop a health promotion programme for a community and ways of evaluating programme effectiveness.

Sleep

When one sleeps, the body undergoes both physical and psychological restoration. Tissues are repaired and psychological rest and renewal, which are necessary for effective memory and intellectual functioning, are accomplished.

Normal sleep consists of non-rapid eye movement sleep (NREM) and rapid eye movement sleep (REM). The rhythm of sleep progresses in a repeating cycle through NREM and REM stages. Each cycle takes approximately 90 minutes to complete, and on a typical night, most people have four to five complete sleep cycles. There are four stages in NREM sleep and another type of sleep in the REM period.

STAGE 1 is a transition between wakefulness and sleep which lasts only a few minutes. The person is relaxed and drowsy, but still slightly aware of the surroundings. In STAGE 2 (which lasts 5 to 20 minutes), thinking decreases as the person begins to drift into actual sleep. The person is not aware of the surroundings but still can be awakened easily. STAGE 3 is considered deep sleep. Muscles relax, the heart rate slows, and body temperature decreases. Stage 4 sleep is similar to Stage 3 sleep, with little body or muscle movement, and the person is difficult to wake. Together, the third and fourth stages of sleep last about 15-30 minutes.

At the end of this time, the person enters rapid eye movement (REM) sleep also known as the PERIOD OF DREAMING. This lasts for about 10 minutes and is a lighter stage of sleep. During REM sleep, the heart and respiratory rate, blood pressure, and basal metabolic rate increase and fluctuate. Skeletal muscle activity and deep tendon reflexes are depressed.

Changes in sleep patterns begin by about age 50 and are most obvious beginning around age 65. As one advances in age, *less time is spent in all stages of sleep, there is almost no stage IV sleep* and *less REM sleep*. Most elderly do not sleep for more than six hours per night, and awaken two to four times per night. They frequently complain of:

- *trouble falling asleep;*
- *trouble staying asleep;*
- *early awakening*; and
- *not feeling rested.*

The causes of the change in sleep patterns are unknown but some suggest that it is due to (1) degeneration of the nervous system or (2) a reduction in cerebral blood flow and an increase in senile plaques within the brain.

In addition to changes in the physiology of the sleep cycle, numerous other factors impair the sleep patterns of older people. Many older people have medical and emotional problems which affect their sleep. Common physical and functional problems include cardiovascular disease, pulmonary disease, snoring, chronic pain from such conditions as arthritis, the side effects of certain medications, and getting up to urinate. Examples of emotional factors would be fear, anxiety and worry, loss of the sleeping partner (because of death). The sleep of older people is also more easily affected by noise, light and chemical stimulants such as coffee and alcohol.

In hospitals and nursing homes or long-term care institutions, sleep patterns of the elderly are effected by additional factors. *Lack of stimulating programmes and activities*, and little conversation sometimes means that they are left to sleep in their rooms or in chairs frequently during the daytime. *Noise* from other residents who are confused, and *institutional schedules* such as taking temperatures, toileting, and giving medications make sleep difficult. The *strangeness of the environment* can keep the elderly awake with fear.

IMPLICATIONS AND RECOMMENDATIONS

The interrupted night-time sleep patterns of older persons can lead to *daytime sleepiness* and *excessive napping*. Two factors contribute to daytime sleepiness: (1) the amount of sleep the night before or for several nights before and (2) the time of day (*there is more sleepiness in the middle of the afternoon* due to circadian rhythms). The observation that elderly people nap throughout the day simply because they are old is *not true*. More likely, they fall asleep frequently in the daytime because the quantity and quality of their night-time sleep has been changed.

Other consequences of interrupted night-time sleep patterns ofthe elderly are *fatigue*, *lack of alertness* leading to *accidents* and *falls, decreased motivation* and *energy* to participate in social and recreational activities and self care, *decreased pain tolerance, irritable* and/or *aggressive* mood, and *depression*.

Assessment of sleep patterns and evaluation of problems should begin with by taking a sleep history. Examples of questions to ask *include "How is your sleep different from previous patterns*?", "Do problems with your sleep interfere with daily functioning?", and "What measures have you taken to try to relieve the problem?" Having the person keep a diary of his/her sleep patterns for several days can be very helpful. In addition to asking about the nature and quality of the sleep, the assessment needs to include questions about all the factors which may be effecting sleep, such as medication usage, respiratory and cardiovascular disease history, and worries. Interventions become more individualized the more specifically the range of problems can be made.

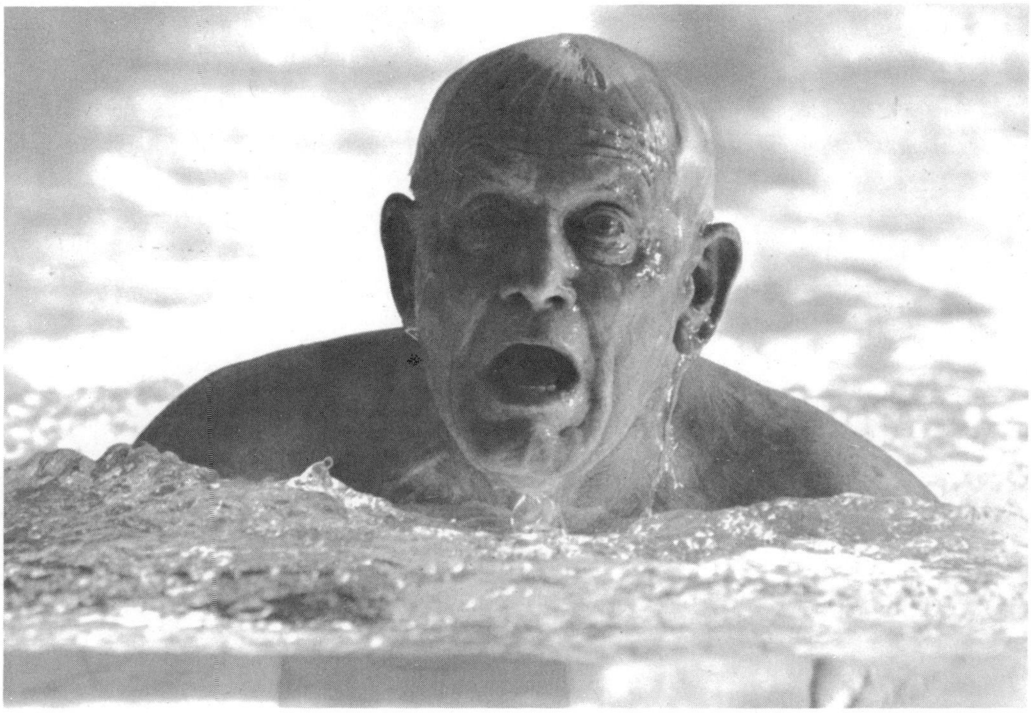

Photo courtesy of David Highet

Regular exercise promotes good sleep and reduces aches.

In all older persons, try to *avoid* the use of *sleeping pills* because changes in the kidneys and liver make the effects of these drugs hard to predict. Sleeping medications tend to accumulate in the body over several days of use, and can cause many more problems than they cure. Use of hypnotics usually only offers short-term relief and can result in (1) impairing daytime functioning by directly affecting daytime alertness and increasing sleep in the daytime, (2) interfering with the ability to sleep the next night, and (3) making chronic conditions such as respiratory disease worse by accumulating in the blood stream.

> It is very important to reinforce good sleep habits in order to overcome age-related changes.

Regular physical exercise such as walking promotes better sleep. The exercise should be done at least two hours *before going to sleep* to avoid stimulation. Naps should be kept to a minimum and discouraged in the early evening. Try to keep the older person engaged in some activity or conversation to get over the early evening sleepy period.

As night-time approaches, do not permit falling asleep in chairs. Just before going to bed, taking a hot bath, receiving a backrub, reading a book or drinking warm milk may help the older person to sleep. *Warm milk may release* **L-tryptophan** which is contained in milk and which has been identified as a sleep inducer. Dim the lights rather than turning them off completely to reduce confusion and possibility of falls. Keep radios, television and conversation away or very quiet. Sleep in loose clothing to allow movement.

If stress or anxiety is a problem, show the older person how to do slow rhythmic breathing, concentrating on air going in and out, imagining a restful scene that evokes relaxing and serene feelings. Yoga and other muscle relaxation techniques should be practised during the day and before going to bed. Praying with the older person and meditation are often helpful as well. Correct wrong expectations and misconceptions about sleep by explaining the changes expected with aging.

If the older person still cannot sleep, they do not have to stay in bed. Instead, they should get up but remain inactive to preserve the rest cycle, and repeat the positive rest measures and return to bed at a later time.

Generally, environmental factors and nursing care routines can be improved. Reducing noise and unnecessary interruptions can usually be done by determining the sources of these. Institutional policies as to when vital signs are taken and medications scheduled can be modified so that they disturb sleep less. Then only clearly necessary procedures such as changing for wetness would need to be done in the night.

Nutrition

Nutritional requirements and guidelines for older adults are very similar to those for younger people. Older people may occasionally need to adhere to recommended dietary intake more vigorously in order to counteract age-related changes or illnesses. More often, the emphasis should be on ensuring that they are eating nutritious and easily digested diet by making food accessible, convenient and tasty.

Reductions in body mass, body metabolism and physical activity lower energy (caloric) needs.

Changes in the *perception* of taste and smell may make food less enjoyable and problems with dentures, lack of teeth or tooth and gum problems may reduce appetite. Other factors which contribute to poor nutrition are decreased exercise, loneliness and depression, chronic illness, dementia (confusion, forgetfulness), the side effects of drugs, alcohol, and smoking. The most prevalent deficiencies may include iron, fibre, folate, vitamin C, calcium, zinc, riboflavin and vitamin A.

Offering small amounts of food frequently can help ensure that adequate amounts are taken. Sometimes removing the upper dentures may permit better taste of food (Staab & Lyles, 1990; Heckheimer, 1989). Use foods which are easily chewed and be certain to have adequate fluid available, since less saliva is secreted and it is thicker.

Many people in hospitals and nursing homes are malnourished. Malnourishment impairs the immune system, increases infection rate, decreases circulating protein and results in poor wound healing, increased mortality, and confusion (especially if dehydration is present).

REMEMBER:	**Family education is very important. Food is a symbol of love and caring and trying to have families avoid certain foods may be in conflict with their caregiving and love. (Staab & Lyles, 1990).**

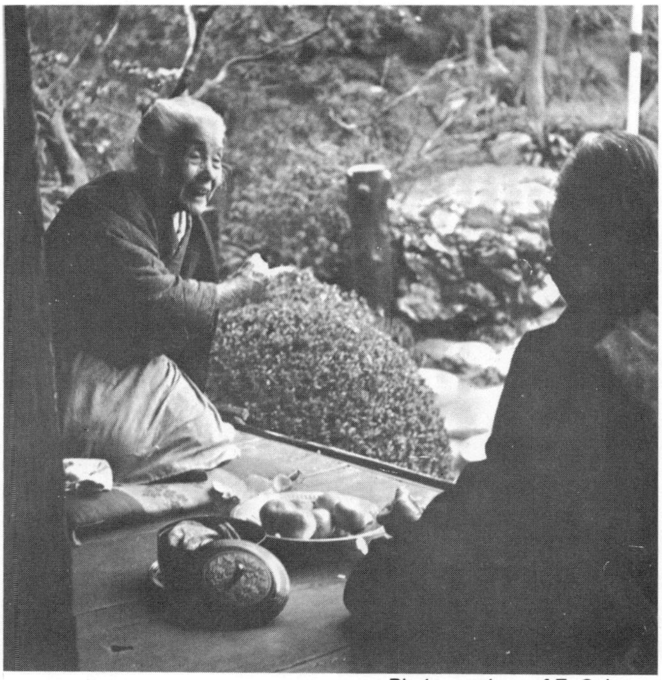

Photo courtesy of E. Schwar

Healthy food is important while love and caring are expressed by sharing of food.

The idea of an " ideal body weight" is only an approximation and depends on activity, genetically defined body type, body composition, ethnicity, and so on. However, as a rough guide, one can take the ideal body weight for men to be equal to or about 49 kg or 106 pounds for the first 153 cm or 5 feet of height plus 1 kg for every cm or 6 pounds for every inch over this; and for women to be about 45 kg or 100 pounds for the first 153 cm or 5 feet plus 1 kg for every cm or 5 pounds for every inch over 153 cm or 5 feet. Ideal weight is typically maintained on a diet of 30 calories per kg of body weight. (Heckheimer, 1989).

In the daily diet there should be at least two servings of milk and milk products, four servings of fruits and vegetables, two servings of meat and meat equivalents, and four servings of grain and grain products. In some cultures, dietary calcium comes from sources other than milk, e.g. small fish bones. A good source of teaching information comes from the SPC/USP series on nutrition for health workers (see references on page 19).

Saturated fat and cholesterol should be *avoided*,

- butter, cream, lard, beef, pork and duck are high in saturated fat. **Monosaturated (e.g. olive oil) and polyunsaturated fats and oils should be used instead**.

- oils made from safflower, sunflower, corn, soy bean, cottonseed, olive, and peanut are good substitutes (although coconut and palm oils are saturated, their hypercholesterolemic effect is still uncertain).

The *goal* of decreasing fat intake is to reduce the formation of atherosclerotic plaques and the likelihood of hypertension and stroke, and probably some cancers.

In addition to diet, exercise and maintenance of reasonable weight help keep cholesterol down.

Animal protein should be *decreased* in most "Western style" diets and plant protein *increased*; fish and chicken should be encouraged in all diets. What constitutes a healthy diet will vary according to what foods are available and culturally acceptable. Most traditional Asian and Pacific diets are now considered to have been close to ideal, at least for adults and the elderly.

Healthy diet pointers*

Remember that plant proteins are *partial proteins*. Two partial proteins must be eaten together to form a complete protein.

- use dried beans, lentils, and nuts for plant proteins.
- cereal with milk, macaroni and cheese, beans plus rice, and a cheese sandwich are examples of how two partial proteins combine to make a complete protein.

Simple carbohydrates should be avoided and complex carbohydrates and fibre should be increased.

- sugar, syrups, colas, and candy are simple carbohydrates.
- bread, cereals such as rice and wheat (especially if not overly processed), root crops such as yam, taro, sweet potatoes, etc., pasta, fruits, vegetables, seeds, beans, and legumes are complex carbohydrates with high fibre content.

Complex, high fibre foods help to lower cholesterol and blood pressure, minimize glucose intolerance and prevent constipation.

Calcium and vitamin D should be ***increased*** to compensate for osteoporotic changes.

- low-fat milk, yogurt, cheese, sardines, certain green vegetables and tofu are high in calcium and vitamin D. Small fish in which the bones are eaten are important sources.

Salt intake should be ***limited*** by substituting herbs, lemon juice, spices, etc. When salt is used it should be iodized.

- canned soups, beans and vegetables, hot dogs, canned meats and meat spreads, ham, bacon, sausage, canned tuna, salmon, sardines, fast foods, processed cheese, baking powder, baking soda, and smoked meat and fish are all high in salt.

*Adapt to local customs

Foods that help protect against cancer

Researchers are finding that what one eats may help block cancer growth by inhibiting the various stages in the cancer process. For example, **antioxidants**, found in some vitamins and minerals, can (1) *eliminate oxygen-free radicals*, substances that seem to make cells more susceptible to cancer, and (2) possibly repair some of the damage to cells that has been done. Wheat bran has been shown to shrink precancerous cells.

One of the most studied antioxidants in vegetables and fruits is **beta-carotene**, which is found in green, yellow and orange *vegetables* such as carrots, sweet potatoes,and spinach and in *fruits* such as apricots and cantaloups.

Lycopene (a red pigment) found in tomatoes and watermelons is another antioxidant. Soybeans contain at least five compounds that are believed to inhibit cancer. Because it is not yet certain which components are most responsible for these positive effects, it is better to recommend eating a varied diet high in fresh fruits and vegetables rather than relying on vitamin supplements. However, vitamin supplements may be used for some elderly people living in inner cities who have difficulty getting fresh fruits and vegetables.

Screening

Regular screening, case-finding and referral should be done for hypertension and cancer (**breast, cervix, colorectal, prostate**).

About 50% of all **breast cancers** occur in women over 65. All women should be instructed in how to do a breast self exam (BSE) and to do it at least every month.

Cancer of the colon and rectum increase with age. Cancer of the colon is more common in women and cancer of the rectum is more common in men. Symptoms include change in bowel habits (new onset constipation or diarrhoea, decreased size of stool or blood in stool), loss of appetite (anorexia), wasting, weight loss, weakness, and dull pain radiating to the back which can be relieved by bending. The mortality associated with this disease is high. Colon/rectal exams are recommended for screening for cancer. Digital rectal exam and examination of stool to check for occult (hidden) blood should be a part of routine health checks for people over 40 years of age. For people over 50 years of age, a proctoscopic examination should be considered every three to five years.

Cancer of the cervix has a peak incidence between 50 and 70 years of age. After 40, all women should have a yearly pelvic examination including a pap smear.

Cancer of the prostate increases with age. It may have no symptoms and as many as one-third may go undetected. All men over 50 years of age should have an annual rectal/digital prostate examination.

REMEMBER: Vision, hearing, teeth, and feet of older people should be inspected periodically.

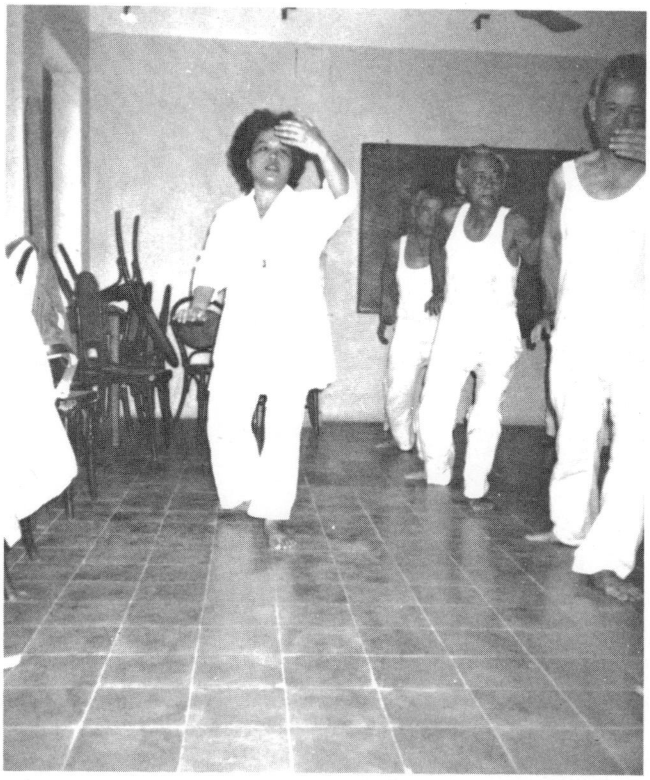

Photo courtesy of Dr Chen Ken

Routine exercises for the elderly are encouraged in China.

Exercise

Regular exercise such as walking should be a part of the daily routine.

One of the oldest methods of preserving health is the practice of performing routine exercises. There are a number of different kinds of body building, breathing, and body movement health preservation exercises which are very beneficial to people of all ages, especially as they get older. It is believed that people who exercise regularly ward off illness, keep fit, and live longer. It is important that the method of exercise and the right type of exercise is chosen. Today, in many communities there are teachers who can provide this type of knowledge, or books can be found which describe exercises for the elderly. It is important to remember that the exercise should be done regularly, It should no be too strenous so that it does not damage an organ, such as the heart, and the older person should feel happy about performing the exercise.

Smoking

Smoking should be eliminated, or if the person cannot quit, at least cut down. Treatment for smoking cessation can include (1) *use of support groups*, (2) *information about the long and short-term effects*, (3) *discussions and films*, (4) *modelling and role-playing of refusal skills* such as, "No thank you I no longer smoke", (5) *techniques for substituting other hand activities*, (6) *ways to avoid temptations* such as visualization of the effects, aversion strategies such as keeping a jar full of cigarette butts, self monitoring (records of when tempted, what was done, what the circumstances were and so on), (7) *stimulus control* (avoiding situations which cause the person to want to smoke), (8) *avoidance of stress* (relaxation techniques), (9) *how to prevent relapse* which is very high and depends on the pattern of smoking which the person had, (10) *dietary instruction about foods that avoid weight gain* or dietary instruction following successful quitting of smoking if weight was gained.

Alcohol

Excessive alcohol intake *increases the potential* for *falls* and other *accidents*, which in turn can *lead to loss of independence* in lifestyle. Reliance on alcohol can *isolate elderly people from needed opportunities for social participation*, increasing feelings of *loneliness* and the risk for *suicide*. Alcohol is a drug which is a depressant *not* a stimulant. Depression and alcohol use often go hand in hand.

Alcohol has practically no nutritional value and over-use of it contributes to *poor nutrition* by (1) reducing proper intake of food during episodes of drinking, and (2) altering the absorption and metabolism of food nutrients. Alcohol can reduce **immune system** response, cause **cardiomyopathies** and **atrophic gastritis**, and aggravate chronic diseases such as **hypertension**.

Discovery of alcohol abuse in older adults is complicated by (1) age-related changes in physiology, (2) the presence of chronic disease, (3) the effects of medications, and (4) differences in role and life-style in the retirement years. As in younger persons who depend on alcohol, *denial* by the elderly and their families is common.

In older persons, the blood level of alcohol necessary to produce the intoxication effect can be achieved with relatively small amounts. There are several explanations for this statement.

- Older persons have decreased total body water, with an increased percentage of body fat. This leads to a greater distribution of fat-soluble substances which require longer time to be eliminated from the body.

- Alcohol slows hepatic metabolism, prolonging and increasing the effect of alcohol.
- Liver enzymes which detoxify alcohol may be less efficient in older persons.
- Blood flow to the liver decreases with age, and this also slows the clearance of alcohol.
- Changes in liver function are accompanied by an apparent increase in brain sensitivity to all central nervous system depressing drugs. Even small amounts of alcohol can bring about mental status changes in older persons.

Symptoms of intoxication and withdrawal *can be easily mistaken* for diseases and age-related physical changes. For example, shakiness caused by drinking may look like senile tremors or Parkinson's disease. Mental status changes brought about by alcohol use can be mistaken for dementing illness.

Intake of alcohol and *the behaviours which one would expect* to occur when alcohol is abused, are often *hard to observe in older persons.* Many elderly (1) spend a lot of time alone so they have greater opportunity to drink alcohol without others seeing, (2) social participation may be less so that drinking patterns are seldom seen outside the home, and (3) may not get loud and argumentative as do some younger persons when they drink, especially if they are frail. Behaviour resulting from intoxication is likely to be passive rather than boisterous.

IMPLICATIONS AND RECOMMENDATIONS

In addition to its direct effect as a drug, alcohol makes the effects of medications unpredictable. During active periods of drinking, alcohol can slow metabolism of drugs by the liver, resulting in increased drug levels. *Long-term* use of alcohol can cause the liver *to accelerate metabolism*, thereby causing drugs to be cleared *prematurely.* Alcohol is especially dangerous in combination with drugs which depress the central nervous system such as sedatives, tricyclic antidepressants, antianxiety drugs, benzodiazepines, neuroleptic drugs, and certain painkillers.

Health care workers are often *not aware* of the alcohol abuse of their older patients. Memory loss, poor balance and frequent falls, may be ignored as being normal consequences of aging. **Stereotypes**, such as believing that persons of higher social status are less likely to be alcoholic, can cause health care workers to NOT suspect alcohol use as the cause of other health problems. Young clinicians may be uncomfortable asking questions about drinking, out of feelings of respect for elders. Some may have the attitude that one should not take away one of the few remaining pleasures available to the elderly.

Drinking problems often must be assessed through indirect methods. Questions should be asked as *to whether the person has a history of falls or accidents*, episodes of *confusion* which come and go, *symptoms of self-neglect* such as weight loss or poor hygiene, or *lack of attention to usual activities* (such as household chores, shopping). The patient and family should be used as information sources.

Evaluation of mood is helpful in suspected abusers, since it is known that alcohol use and depression are related. The Geriatric Depression Scale (GDS) which was described in Module 10 could be used. Exploration of mood and mental outlook may lead to a fuller and more complete discussion of underlying problems and their relationship to drinking.

If drinking cannot be controlled (that is limited to small, infrequent amounts), it should be stopped completely. If the older person needs to be in hospital, the alcohol treatment usually includes prescription of vitamins, especially thiamine, nutrition, hydration and treatment of withdrawal symptoms.

For withdrawal symptoms, long-acting benzodiazepines as a rule are not given; short to intermediate-acting benzodiazepines are used such as lorazepam (Ativan), and oxazepam (Serax, Bienenfeld) and the doses of these are about one-half what would be given for younger persons. Disulfiram (Antabuse) is seldom used since the way the drug works often poses risks to the cardiovascular system of the elderly.

Withdrawal in elderly may be more *severe* and may *last longer,* and *improvement in mental status and emotional state may resolve more slowly*.

After hospitalization, older alcohol abusers require ongoing support. Referral to community resources including mental health specialists will be needed. Group therapy usually focuses on age-related losses, boredom, loneliness, poor self-esteem, re-engaging the person in social interaction, and problem-solving for other factors which led to the drinking.

Accident prevention

Beyond the obvious issue of the pain and trauma at the time of an injury, the biggest long-term danger is that an injury to an older person is much more likely to result in *immobility* and *loss of function* and possibly lead to greater *complications.* Falls and burns are the most frequent accidents.

A very large number of accidents can be avoided by recognizing and compensating for normal age-related changes. These include changes in vision, hearing, proprioceptor touch, balance and gait, coordination and strength, and temperature regulation. Be especially careful for elderly who are confused, have chronic illnesses such as cardiac arrythmias, those who get postural hypotension, and those who may have side-effects from their medications.

There is a growing body of evidence now to support the observation that when people are under emotional stress they are more susceptible to accidents.

Be constantly alert to the need to anticipate safety needs and create a safe environment.

Use colours which enhance the older person's vision, and use colour to improve depth perception. Remove obstacles, keep the environment well lighted, use only sturdy flat shoes, place stable things (within reach) to hold onto, mark switches in large bold letters for "on" and "off" and so on.

Medication management

As a review, remember that as one ages:

- less gastric acid is secreted;
- the liver function is reduced;
- the kidneys filter only about half as much as in younger years;
- there is less muscle mass and less total body water; and
- there is at least some altered receptor sensitivity.

This results in **absorption, metabolism and excretion** of medications being:

- altered;
- less predictable than for younger persons;
- often having an additive effect; and
- frequently having adverse side effects.

Common drug classes which produce adverse reactions are antibiotics, antiarrythmics such as digoxin, diuretics, anti-Parkinsonian agents, cholinergics, sedative-hypnotics, antidepressants, antihypertensives, coumadin, and drugs used to control symptoms in dementia (antipsychotic agents).

Interventions should include:

- frequent review of medications;
- instructions about possible side effects;

minimising the number of drugs used; and

being constantly alert to the fact that, in older persons, medications are often the cause of:

- confusion/dementia
- orthostatic hypotension and falls
- anxiety
- problems with sleep
- constipation
- urinary retention.

Immunizations for older people should include at least **Tetanus Toxoid** and **Hepatitis B** vaccines.

Concluding points

1. Many assessment instruments are available for health screening of older people. However, few of these have been evaluated using back translation techniques. That is, the meaning that the questions may have in one language (the language in which it was developed) may be substantially different from the meaning in another language. Some instruments appear to have more consistency in wording than others. The ones which have been included in the various modules are suggested for use with understanding of their limitations cross-culturally. Another standard assessment instrument for determining functional status, The Barthel Index, is included in this module on pages 17-18. Until more research is done on the cross-cultural validity of these screening tools, the usefulness of them is not known. Clinical judgement based on good interviewing techniques and knowledge of age-related normal changes is always a good approach.

2. Physical health is very important to the energy and adaptive ability of older persons. (Butler & Lewis, 1977). Preventive practices and early intervention support the physical and emotional well-being of elderly persons.

3. Symptoms of illness in elderly persons are often *unusual, vague* and/or *nonspecific.* Infections such as pneumonia and urinary tract infections may be present without accompanying fever. Confusion may be a symptom of pneumonia, sodium loss, depression or many other conditions. With myocardial infarction (heart attacks), the chest pain may be mild instead of crushing. Older persons may have hyperactivity (be agitated) with depression rather than lethargy. (Bender, 1992; Rosenthal & Rosenthal, 1990; Fox, 1988).

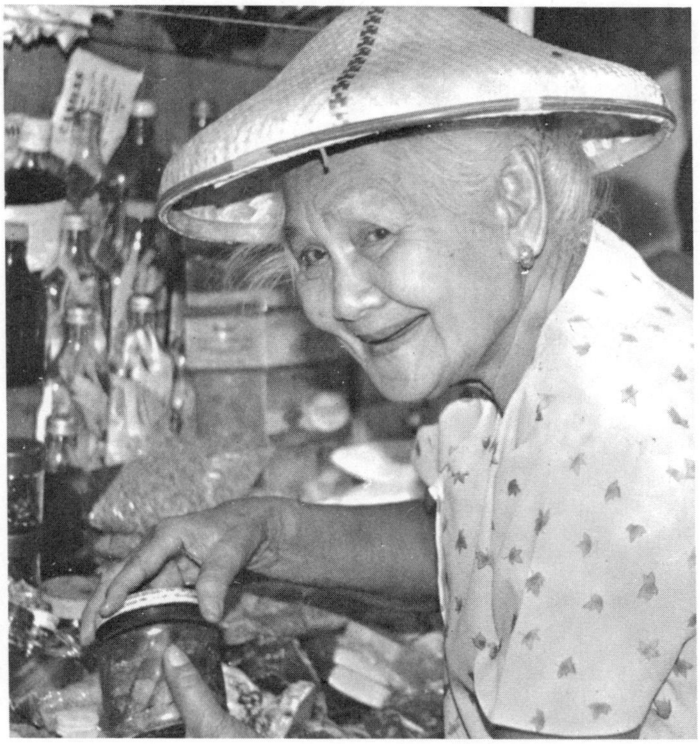

Photo courtesy of T. Miller

Physical health is very important to the energy and adaptive ability of older persons. This Filipina elderly drinks herbal tea for cleansing the urinary system.

4. It is very important that the elderly are given the ability to find solutions to their health problems and use their own skills in implementing these behaviours. Samples of messages that will help the older person to stay healthy are given in the brochure in the pocket at the end of this manual. These were prepared by the Health Promotion Unit, WHO, Western Pacific Regional Office.

Exercise A

Enact the following situation in a role-play. Mrs. L is 45 years old and has been taking care of her 70-year old mother for three years. Lately the mother has been up most nights and napping throughout the day. Mrs. L is very upset because she is not getting much sleep herself. She tells you that if something is not done to help her soon, she will be too tired to keep her daytime job (she cannot afford to lose it). Propose factors that need to be assessed. Develop a plan for this family, including education about the normal age-related changes in the sleep-wake cycle.

Exercise B

The local department of health needs to have a programme developed for immunization and cancer screening for older people. As a group, develop the plan including specific immunization programmes needed and specific cancer screens needed. How do you intend to let people know about it? How will you know if it has been effective? What kinds of teaching need to be done for the older people and possibly their families?

Short-answer exercise

1. Explain how you would go about implementing some of the approaches which were suggested to help older persons quit smoking.

2. All older women should be performing breast self exam (BSE) on themselves monthly. How do you go about teaching this important self exam? Jot down some ideas about the approach you might use.

3. Briefly describe why medications are such an important consideration in monitoring the health of older adults.

Suggested field experience for assessment of practical skills

This can be done in almost any setting where there are older adults. Students can use the list in the Assessment of Practical Skills section of this manual and develop plans of care. The Barthel Instrument follows on the next two pages and this would be interesting for them to use as well.

Name ____________________ Date of Evaluation ____________

BARTHEL INDEX

1. Feeding - Can the patient feed self a meal from a tray or table when someone puts the food within reach. They must put on an assistive device if this is needed, cut food, use salt and pepper, spread butter, etc. Patient must accomplish this in a reasonable time.
   10 = Independent
   5 = Some help is necessary (with cutting up food, etc. as listed above).

2. Moving - Patients can safely approach the bed in a wheelchair, lock brakes, lift footrests, move safely to bed, lie down, come to a sitting position on the side of the bed, change the position of the wheelchair, if necessary, to transfer back into it safely, and return to the wheelchair.
   15 = Independent in all phases of this activity
   10 = Either some minimal help is needed in some step of this activity or the patient needs to be reminded or supervised for safety of one or more parts of this activity.
   5 = Patient can come to a sitting position without the help of a second person but needs to be lifted out of bed, or if a great deal of help is needed in transfer.

3. Personal toilet - Patient can wash hands and face, comb hair, clean teeth, and shave. He may use any kind of razor but must put in blade or plug in razor without help as well as get it from drawer or cabinet. Female patients must put on own make-up, if used, but need not braid or style her hair.
   5 = Independent

4. Getting on and off toilet - Patient is able to get on and off toilet, fasten and unfasten clothes, prevent soiling of clothes, and use toilet paper without help. A wall bar or other stable object may be used for support if needed. If it is necessary to use a bed pan instead of a toilet, patient must be able to place it on a chair, emply, and clean it.
   10 = Independent
   5 = Patient needs help because of imbalance or in handling clothes or in using toilet paper.

5. Bathing self - Patient may use a bath tub, shower, or take a complete sponge bath. Patient must be able to do all the steps involved in whichever method is employed without another person being present.
   5 = Independent

Ask either question 6 if the patient walks or 6a if a wheelchair is used but do not ask both.

6. Walking on a level surface - Patient can walk at least 50 yards without help or supervision. Patient may wear braces or prostheses and use crutches, canes, or a walkerette but not a rolling walker. They must be able to lock and unlock brakes if used, assume the standing position and sit down, get the necessary mechanical aides into position for use, and dispose of them when sitting.
   15 = Independent
   10 = Patient needs help or supervision in any of the above but can walk at least 50 yards with a little help.

6a. Propelling a wheelchair - If a patient cannot ambulate but can propel a wheelchair independently. Patient must be able to go around corners, turn around, maneuver the chair to a table, bed, toilet, etc. They must be able to push at least 50 yards.
   5 = Independent

7. Ascending and descending stairs - Patient is able to go up and down a flight of stairs safely without help or supervision. They may and should use handrails, canes, or

crutches when needed, and must be able to carry canes or crutches ascending or descending stairs.
10 = Independent
5 = Patient needs help with or supervision of any of the above items.

8. <u>Dressing and undressing</u> - Patient is able to put on and remove and fasten all clothing, and tie shoe laces (unless it is necessary to use adaptations for this). The activity includes putting on and removing fastening corset or braces when these are prescribed. Special clothing such as suspenders, loafer shoes, dresses that open down the front may be used when necessary.
10 = Independent
5 = Patient needs help in putting on and removing or fastening any clothing. They must do at least half the work themselves. Task must be accomplished in a reasonable time. Women need not be scored on use of a brassiere or girdle unless these are prescribed garments.

9. <u>Continence of bowels</u> - Patient is able to control bowels and have no accidents. They can use a suppository or take an enema when necessary (as for spinal cord injury patients who have had bowel training).
10 = Independent
5 = Patient needs help in using a suppository or taking an enema or has occasional accidents.

10. <u>Controlling bladder</u> - Patient is able to control bladder day and night. Spinal cord injury patients who wear an external device and leg bag put them on independently, clean and empty bag, and stay dry day and night.
10 = Independent
5 = Patient has occasional accidents or cannot wait for bed pan or get to the toilet in time or needs help with an external device.

____Total Score (lowest score possible 0; highest score possible 100)

Mahoney, F.I. & Barthel, D.W. (1965). Functional evaluation: The Barthel index. <u>Maryland State Medical Journal</u>, 14, 61-65.

Bibliography

Exercise, nutrition, cancer screening, accident prevention, medication management

Alcorn, J.M. (1992). Colorectal cancer prevention: A primary care approach. Geriatrics, 47(2): 24-30.

Alford, D.M. (1991). Tips on promoting food and fluid intake in the elderly. Journal of Gerontological Nursing. 17(11): 44-46.

Blocker, W.P. (1992). Maintaining functional independence by mobilizing the aged. Geriatrics, 47(1): 48-20, 53.

Campbell, A.J. (1991). Drug treatment as a cause of falls in old age. A review of the offending agents. Drugs and Aging. 1(4): 289-302.

Carnevali, D.L. & Patrick, M. (Eds.)(1993). Nursing management for the elderly (3rd ed.). Philadelphia: J.B. Lippincott.

Fisher, M. (Ed.)(1989). Guide to clinical preventive services: An assessment of the effectiveness of 169 interventions (Report of the US Preventive Services Task Force). Baltimore, MD: Williams & Wilkins

Fleischer, D. E. et al. (1989). Detection and surveillance of colorectal cancer. Journal of the American Medical Association, 262(4), 580-585.

Fox, R.A. (1988). Atypical presentation of geriatric infections. Geriatrics, 43(5), 58-59, 6-64, 68.

Frank-Stromborg, M. & Olsen, S.J. (1993). Cancer prevention in minority populations: Cultural implications for health care professionals. St. Louis: Mosby.

Grimley, E.J. (1992). Medication, fallers and non-fallers. Age/Ageing, 21(3): 226-227.

Hale, W.A. (1992). Characteristics and predictors of falls in elderly patients. Journal of Family Practitioners, 34(5): 577-581.

Heckheimer, E.F. (1989). Health promotion of the elderly in the community. Philadelphia: W.B. Saunders.

Horwath, C.C. (1991). Nutrition goals for older adults: A review. The Gerontologist, 31(6): 811-821.

Kane, R.L., Ouslander, J.G. & Abrass, I.B.(1984). Essentials of clinical geriatrics. New York: McGraw-Hill.

Keintz, M.K., Rimer, B., Fleisher, L., & Engstrom, P. (1988). Educating older adults about their increased cancer risk. The Gerontologist, 28(4): 487-887.

Lieberman, D.A. (1990). Colon cancer screening. Archives of Internal Medicine, 150(April): 740-744.

Robie, P.W. (1989). Cancer screening in the elderly. Journal of American Geriatrics Society, 37(9): 888-893.

Rosenthal, G., & Rosenthal, S.K. (1990). Differences in presentation of Disease. Principles of Geriatric Medicine and Gerontology.

Sennott-Miller, L., & Kligman, E.W. (1992). Healthier lifestyle: How to motivate older patients to change. Geriatrics, 47(12): 52-56, 58-59.

South Pacific Community Nutrition Training Project series (1990). University of the South Pacific: Suva, Fiji.

Tessier, M-C, Rosario, D.B., Finau, S., Malolo, M., Dignan, C.., Terrel-Perico, S. & Cieniembo, B.K. (1993). Prevention of non-communicable diseases in the Pacific training module for social mobilization and community action. Handbook no. 42. South Pacific Commission.

Wood, L. (1992). Fall risk protocol and nursing care plan. Geriatric Nursing, 13(4): 205-206.

Sleep

Ancoli-Israeli, S. Parker, L. & Kripke, D.F. (1989). Sleep fragmentation in patients from a nursing home. Journal of Gerontology, 44: 18-21.

Brody, & Vijajashankar. (1977). Anatomical changes in the nervous system. In C.E. Finch & L. Hayflick (Eds). Handbook of the biology of aging. (pp. 241-261), New York: Van Norstrand Reinhold.

Carskadon, M. (1990). Daytime sleepiness: Clinical consequences and treatment. National Institutes of Health Consensus Conference, abstract, p. 83.

Carskadon, M.A. & Dement, W.C. (1985). Sleep loss in elderly volunteers. Sleep, 8(3): 207-221.

Clapin-French, E. (1986). Sleep patterns of aged persons in long-term care facilities. Journal of Advanced Nursing, 11: 57-66.

Consensus Conference (1990). The treatment of sleep disorders of older people. National Institutes of Health, Bethesda, Maryland, USA.

Crosby, L. (1994). Personal communication. University of Arizona, College of Nursing, Tucson, Arizona 85721.

Dement, W., Miles, L.E. & Carskadon, M.A. (1992). White paper in sleep and aging. Journal of the American Geriatrics Society, 30: 25-50.

Friedman, L., Bliwise, D.L., Yesavage, J.A. & Salom, S.R. (1991). A preliminary study comparing sleep restriction and relaxation treatments for insomnia in older adults. Journal of Gerontology, 46(1): p1-8.

Hoch, C. & Reynolds, C. (1986). Sleep disturbances and what to do about them. Geriatric Nursing, (January/February):24-27.

Jacobs, D., Ancoli-Israel, S., Parker, L. & Kripke, D.F. (1989). Twenty-four sleep-wake pattrns in a nursing home population. Psychology & Aging, 4: 352-356.

Johnson, D. & Crosby, L. (1991). Subjective evaluation of sleep in longterm care facility. Unpublished master's thesis, University of Arizona College of Nursing, Tucson, Arizona, USA.

Karacan, I. & Williams, R.L. (1983). Sleep disorders in the elderly. American Family Physician, 27(3): 143-152.

Alcohol

Allen, J.P., Eckardt, M. J. & Wallen, J. (1988). Screening for alcoholism: Techniques and issues. Public Health Reports, 103(6): 586-592.

Beck, A.T., Steer, R.A. & Trexler, L.D. (1989). Alcohol abuse and eventual suicide: A 5 - to 10-year prospective of alcohol-abusing attempters. Journal of Studies on Alcohol, 50(3): 202-209.

Bienenfeld, D. (1990). Substance abuse. In D. Bienenfeld (Ed.), Verwoerdt's clinical geropsychiatry (pp. 164-177). Baltimore: Williams & Wilkens.

Brown, B.B. (1982). Professionals' perceptions of drug and alcohol abuse among the elderly. The Gerontologist, 22(6): 519-525.

Closser, M.H. (1991). Benzodiazepines and the elderly: A review of potential problems. Journal of Substance Abuse Treatment, 8(1): 35-41.

Curtis, J.R., Geller, G., Stokes, E.J., Levine, D.M. & Moore, R.D. (1989). Characteristics, diagnosis, and treatment of alcoholism in elderly patients. Journal of the American Geriatrics Society, 37(4): 310-316.

Gomberg, E.S. (1990). Drugs, alcohol and aging. In L.T. Kozlowski, H.M. Annis, H.D. Cappell, F.B. Glaser, M.S. Goodstadt, Y. Israel, H. Kalant, E.M. Sellers & E.R. Vingilis (Eds.), Research advances in alcohol and drug problems (pp. 171-214). New York: Plenum Press.

Gruchow, H.W., Barboriak, J.J. & Sobocinski, K.A. (1989). Alcohol consumption and abuse among women and the elderly. In R.R. Watson (Ed.), Diagnosis of alcohol abuse (pp. 217-230). Boca Raton, FL: CRC Press.

Hartford, J.T. & Samorajski, T. (1982). Alcoholism in the geriatric population. Journal of the American Geriatrics Society, 30(1): 18-24.

Hingson, R. & Howland, J. (1987). Alcohol as a risk factor from accidental falls: A review of the literature. Journal of Studies on Alcohol, 48(3): 212-219.

Jacobson, G.R. (1989). Identification of problem drinkers and alcoholics. In R.R. Watson (Ed.), Diagnosis of alcohol abuse (pp. 177-200). Boca Raton, FL: CRC Press.

Mackel, C., Sheehy, C. & Badger, T. (1994). The challenge of detection and treatment of alcohol abuse among elders. Clinical Nurse Specialist, accepted for publication in the 8(4) issue.

Metzger, D.S. & O'Brien, C.P. (1990). Substance abuse: The challenge of assessment. In B. Spilker (Ed.), Quality of life assessments in clinical trials (pp. 237-246). New York: Raven Press.

Miller, N.S. (1990). Alcohol and drug dependence. In J. Sadavoy, L.W. Lazarus & L.F. Jarvick (Eds.) Comprehensive Review of Geriatric Psychiatry (pp. 387-401). Washington DC: American Psychiatric Press.

Mohs, M.E. & Watson, R.R. (1989a). Changes in nutrient status and balance associated with alcohol abuse. In R.R. Watson (Ed.), Diagnosis of alcohol abuse (pp. 125-146). Boca Raton, FL: CRC Press.

Mohs, M.E. & Watson, R.R. (1989b). Changes in enzymes and other biochemical markers associated with alcohol abuse. In R.R. Watson (Ed.), Diagnosis of alcohol abuse (pp. 69-100). Boca Raton, Fl: CRC Press.

Pruzinsky, E.W. (1987). Alcohol and the elderly, Journal of Gerontological Social Work, 11(1): 81-93.

Schuckit, M.A. (1982). A clinical review of alcohol, alcoholism, and the elderly patient. Journal of Clinical Psychiatry, 43(10): 396-399.

Scott, R.B. & Mitchell, M.C. (1988). Aging, alcohol and the liver. Journal of the American Geriatric Society, 36(3): 255-265.

Sheikh, J.I. & Yesavage, J.A. (1986). Geriatric Depression Scale (GDS): Recent evidence and development of a shorter version. Clinical Gerontology, 5(1/2): 165-172.

Shinn, A.F. & Shrewsbury, R.P. (Eds.). (1985). Evaluations of drug interactions. (3rd ed.). St. Louis: CV Mosby.

Stinson, F.S., DuFour, M.C. & Bertolucci, D. (1989). Epidemiological bulletin No. 20: Alcohol-related morbidity in the aging population. Alcohol Health & Research World, 13(1): 80-87.

Subcommittee on Health and Long-Term Care. (1992). Alcohol abuse and misuse among the elderly. (Committee Publication. No. 102-852, USGPO). Washington, DC: U.S. Government Printing Office.

Thienhaus, O.J. & Hartford, J.T. (1984). Alcoholism in the elderly. Psychiatric Medicine, 2(1): 27-41.

Vestal, R.E., McGuire, E.A., Tobin, J.D., Andres, R., Norris, A.H. & Mezey, E. (1977). Aging and ethanol metabolism. Clinical Pharmacology and Therapeutics, 21(3): 343-354.

Annexes

STUDENT EVALUATION TOOLS

Assessment of Practical Skills

Module 2 - The senses

Student's Name: ______________________ Instructor's Name ____________________

Date of Clinical Experience: ____

Simulation Exercise: ____

Healthcare Setting: ____

EVALUATE THE STUDENT'S PERFORMANCE BY SCORING EACH ITEM USING THE FOLLOWING CRITERIA:

Superior: Accurate performance with minimal supervision and clarification needed.
Satisfactory: Accurate performance with occassional supervision and clarification needed.
Unsatisfactory: Frequent inaccuracies in performance and frequent clarification needed.

	Superior	Satisfactory	Unsatisfactory
CLINICAL ASSESSMENT SKILLS			
1. Notes distribution and location of fat and muscle, and joints that are prominent.			
2. Checks skin tone (turgor) by gently pinching skin and lifting up; observes for changes in pigmentation including *lentigo senilis* and for dryness.			
3. Observes changes in hair colour and notes hair loss on head, chest and/or other appropriate locations.			
4. Recognizes *arcus senilis* and *senile ptosis*.			
5. Checks vision with pocket Snellen chart; checks ability of the older person to see colours.			
6. Observes for dryness and irritation in the eyes.			
7. Asks questions which give clues about visual problems.			
8. Checks hearing using the Shore (1978) method for words: smart, off, with, that, thin, will, cat, room, all, jaw, does.			
9. Consults with appropriate health care worker for evaluating ear wax.			
10. Asks questions which give clues about hearing problems.			
11. Performs checks of smell by having the older person close the eyes and identify peanut butter, cloves, oranges, coffee or other strong scents.			

12. Performs checks of taste by having the older person close the eyes and identify flavoured substances of sugar, salt, mint, lemon juice or other strong tastes.			
13. Asks questions which give clues about problems with taste and smell.			
14. Performs checks of touch with cotton, pin prick and other coarse materials or other fabrics.			
15. Observes the older person's walking gait and draws conclusions.			
16. Asks questions which give clues about problems with sensation and balance.			
17. Consults with appropriate health care workers about problems with cataracts, glaucoma, macula degeneration and diabetic retinopathy.			
18. Uses effective communication skills such as open-ended questions and places the older person at ease; draws conclusions about non-verbal communication of the older person from such things as body language.			
Comments:			
DEVELOPING THE PLAN OF CARE			
1. Assessment data gained in the clinical assessment is comprehensive.			
2. Makes correct nursing diagnoses for actual or potential problems.			
3. Writes goals which are realistic, measurable and written in terms of the older person's accomplishment.			
4. Develops creative nursing interventions for all nursing diagnoses/problems.			
5. Describes the priority of all nursing diagnoses/problems.			
6. Care plans include safety, health promotion and education of the older person.			
Comments:			

General comments and recommendations:

STUDENT EVALUATION TOOLS

Assessment of Practical Skills

Module 3 - The musculoskeletal system

Student's Name: ____________________ Instructor's Name ____________________

Date of Clinical Experience: ____________________

Simulation Exercise: ____________________

Healthcare Setting: ____________________

EVALUATE THE STUDENT'S PERFORMANCE BY SCORING EACH ITEM USING THE FOLLOWING CRITERIA:

Superior: Accurate performance with minimal supervision and clarification needed.
Satisfactory: Accurate performance with occassional supervision and clarification needed.
Unsatisfactory: Frequent inaccuracies in performance and frequent clarification needed.

	Superior	Satisfactory	Unsatisfactory
CLINICAL ASSESSMENT SKILLS			
1. Notes distribution and location of fat and muscle, and movement of joints			
2. Asks questions about menopause (if female), smoking, alcohol use, exercise level and type, calcium intake, and steroid use to estimate risk of osteoporosis.			
3. Observes spine for *kyphosis*.			
4. Observes the older person's walking gait and draws conclusions.			
5. Inspects joints for signs and symptoms of *osteoarthritis* (for example swelling, limitation or pain with movement, crepitus.			
6. Asks questions which give clues related to falls and fractures.			
7. Asks questions which give clues about ability to manage self-care activities.			
8. Reviews medication use in regard to the musculoskeletal system.			
Comments:			

DEVELOPING THE PLAN OF CARE			
1. Assessment data gained in the clinical assessment is comprehensive.			
2. Makes correct nursing diagnoses for actual or potential problems.			
3. Writes goals which are realistic, measurable and written in terms of the older person's accomplishment.			
4. Develops creative nursing interventions for all nursing diagnoses/problems.			
5. Describes the priority of all nursing diagnoses/problems.			
6. Care plans include safety, health promotion and education of the older person.			
Comments:			

General comments and recommendations:

STUDENT EVALUATION TOOLS

Assessment of Practical Skills

Module 4 - The urinary system

Student's Name: ____________________ Instructor's Name ____________________

Date of Clinical Experience: ____________________

Simulation Exercise: ____________________

Healthcare Setting: ____________________

EVALUATE THE STUDENT'S PERFORMANCE BY SCORING EACH ITEM USING THE FOLLOWING CRITERIA:

Superior: Accurate performance with minimal supervision and clarification needed.
Satisfactory: Accurate performance with occassional supervision and clarification needed.
Unsatisfactory: Frequent inaccuracies in performance and frequent clarification needed.

	Superior	Satisfactory	Unsatisfactory
CLINICAL ASSESSMENT SKILLS			
1. Asks questions about urinary bladder status including amount of fluid intake, urine leakage, difficulty initiating the stream, urinary tract infections, history of childbirths (if female), prostate problems (if male), nocturia, timing and surrounding circumstances if urinary leakage exists and so on.			
2. Asks questions about strategies-approaches used by the older person to handle wetness, skin care, odour and so on.			
3. Reviews medication use, especially anticholinergics and diuretics.			
4. Correctly identifies type of urinary incontinence (if any exists).			
5. (if appropriate) Demonstrates KEGEL exercises and has the older person return the demonstration.			
6. (if appropriate) Demonstrates CREDE manoeuvre and has the older person return the demonstration.			
7. Assesses whether urine tests such as routine urine analysis or culture and sensitivity should be done.			
8. Reviews medication use in regard to the urinary system			

9. Consults with apropriate health care worker about problems which require further assessment and treatment.			
Comments:			
DEVELOPING THE PLAN OF CARE			
1. Assessment data gained in the clinical assessment is comprehensive.			
2. Makes correct nursing diagnoses for actual or potential problems.			
3. Writes goals which are realistic, measurable and written in terms of the older person's accomplishment.			
4. Develops creative nursing interventions for all nursing diagnoses/problems.			
5. Describes the priority of all nursing diagnoses/problems.			
6. Care plans include safety, health promotion and education of the older person.			
Comments:			

General comments and recommendations:

STUDENT EVALUATION TOOLS

Assessment of Practical Skills

Module 5 - The gastrointestinal system

Student's Name: ____________________ Instructor's Name ____________________

Date of Clinical Experience: ______________________________

Simulation Exercise: ______________________________

Healthcare Setting: ______________________________

EVALUATE THE STUDENT'S PERFORMANCE BY SCORING EACH ITEM USING THE FOLLOWING CRITERIA:

Superior: Accurate performance with minimal supervision and clarification needed.
Satisfactory: Accurate performance with occassional supervision and clarification needed.
Unsatisfactory: Frequent inaccuracies in performance and frequent clarification needed.

	Superior	Satisfactory	Unsatisfactory
CLINICAL ASSESSMENT SKILLS			
1. Inspects the mouth and teeth.			
2. Interviews about dietary history and asks questions about dietary habits including intake or fibre.			
3. Asks questions about bowel habits, exercise patterns, fluid intake, need for functional assistance, problems with privacy; if a problem exists with constipation, asks what the older person does to manage the problem (such as laxatives, enemas, hot drinks and so on).			
4. Determines whether digital rectal exam and stool checks for hidden blood have been done within the past year.			
5. Reviews medication use in regard to side effects which can cause constipation.			
6. Interviews with the Elimination Instrument and with the Nutrition Screen Level I and II if appropriate.			
7. Asks about change in stool patterns or characteristics.			
8. (for male elderly) Asks about rectal examinations to check for prostate cancer.			

9. Consults with appropriate health care worker about problems with hiatal hernia, cancer of the colon or rectum.			
Comments:			
DEVELOPING THE PLAN OF CARE			
1. Assessment data gained in the clinical assessment is comprehensive.			
2. Makes correct nursing diagnoses for actual or potential problems.			
3. Writes goals which are realistic, measurable and written in terms of the older person's accomplishment.			
4. Develops creative nursing interventions for all nursing diagnoses/problems.			
5. Describes the priority of all nursing diagnoses/problems.			
6. Care plans include safety, health promotion and education of the older person.			
Comments:			

General comments and recommendations:

STUDENT EVALUATION TOOLS

Assessment of Practical Skills

Module 6 - Cardiovascular and respiratory systems

Student's Name: ______________________ Instructor's Name ____________________

Date of Clinical Experience: ____

Simulation Exercise: ____

Healthcare Setting: ____

EVALUATE THE STUDENT'S PERFORMANCE BY SCORING EACH ITEM USING THE FOLLOWING CRITERIA:

Superior: Accurate performance with minimal supervision and clarification needed.
Satisfactory: Accurate performance with occassional supervision and clarification needed.
Unsatisfactory: Frequent inaccuracies in performance and frequent clarification needed.

	Superior	Satisfactory	Unsatisfactory
CLINICAL ASSESSMENT SKILLS			
1. Notes blood pressure and pulse and decides whether they are within normal limits; listens to lungs (breath sounds).			
2. Asks questions related to orthostatic hypotension, falls, dizziness and so on.			
3. Asks questions about smoking, use of alcohol, fat and salt in the diet, use of soluble bran, exercise and health promotion behaviours.			
4. Reviews medications.			
5. Consults with appropriate health care worker about pneumonia, chronic obstructive lung disease and asthma.			
Comments:			

DEVELOPING THE PLAN OF CARE			
1. Assessment data gained in the clinical assessment is comprehensive.			
2. Makes correct nursing diagnoses for actual or potential problems.			
3. Writes goals which are realistic, measurable and written in terms of the older person's accomplishment.			
4. Develops creative nursing interventions for all nursing diagnoses/problems.			
5. Describes the priority of all nursing diagnoses/problems.			
6. Care plans include safety, health promotion and education of the older person.			
Comments:			

General comments and recommendations:

STUDENT EVALUATION TOOLS

Assessment of Practical Skills

Module 7 - Age-related changes in the reproductive system and late life sexuality

Student's Name: ______________________ Instructor's Name ____________________

Date of Clinical Experience: ____

Simulation Exercise: ____

Healthcare Setting: ____

EVALUATE THE STUDENT'S PERFORMANCE BY SCORING EACH ITEM USING THE FOLLOWING CRITERIA:

Superior: Accurate performance with minimal supervision and clarification needed.
Satisfactory: Accurate performance with occassional supervision and clarification needed.
Unsatisfactory: Frequent inaccuracies in performance and frequent clarification needed.

	Superior	Satisfactory	Unsatisfactory
CLINICAL ASSESSMENT SKILLS			
1. For women, asks questions about toileting patterns and problems, number of childbirths, vaginal itching or discharge			
2. For men, asks questions about toileting patterns and problems, and prostate problems.			
3. Consults with appropriate health care workers.			
4. Determines whether (for men and women respectively) prostate, breast and pap checks have been done within the past year.			
Comments:			

DEVELOPING THE PLAN OF CARE			
1. Assessment data gained in the clinical assessment is comprehensive.			
2. Makes correct nursing diagnoses for actual or potential problems.			
3. Writes goals which are realistic, measurable and written in terms of the older person's accomplishment.			
4. Develops creative nursing interventions for all nursing diagnoses/problems.			
5. Describes the priority of all nursing diagnoses/problems.			
6. Care plans include safety, health promotion and education of the older person.			
Comments:			

General comments and recommendations:

STUDENT EVALUATION TOOLS

Assessment of Practical Skills

Module 8 - Endocrine and immune function

Student's Name: ____________________ Instructor's Name ____________________

Date of Clinical Experience: ____________________

Simulation Exercise: ____________________

Healthcare Setting: ____________________

EVALUATE THE STUDENT'S PERFORMANCE BY SCORING EACH ITEM USING THE FOLLOWING CRITERIA:

Superior: Accurate performance with minimal supervision and clarification needed.
Satisfactory: Accurate performance with occassional supervision and clarification needed.
Unsatisfactory: Frequent inaccuracies in performance and frequent clarification needed.

	Superior	Satisfactory	Unsatisfactory
CLINICAL ASSESSMENT SKILLS			
1. Interviews for history of pneumonia, infections and cancer.			
2. Asks questions about exercise level, family history of diabetes, signs and symptoms of diabetes (thirst, fatigue, confusion, weight loss, blurred vision, muscle weakness, itching without presence of a rash); takes weight.			
3. Tests urine for sugar and acetone (if appropriate).			
4. Inspects lower extremeties for vascular flow problems.			
5. Reviews medications.			

Comments:

DEVELOPING THE PLAN OF CARE			
1. Assessment data gained in the clinical assessment is comprehensive.			
2. Makes correct nursing diagnoses for actual or potential problems.			
3. Writes goals which are realistic, measurable and written in terms of the older person's accomplishment.			
4. Develops creative nursing interventions for all nursing diagnoses/problems.			
5. Describes the priority of all nursing diagnoses/problems.			
6. Care plans include safety, health promotion and education of the older person.			
Comments:			

General comments and recommendations:

STUDENT EVALUATION TOOLS

Assessment of Practical Skills

Module 9 - Dementing illness and changes in the brain

Student's Name: ______________________ Instructor's Name ____________________

Date of Clinical Experience: ____

Simulation Exercise: ____

Healthcare Setting: ____

EVALUATE THE STUDENT'S PERFORMANCE BY SCORING EACH ITEM USING THE FOLLOWING CRITERIA:

Superior: Accurate performance with minimal supervision and clarification needed.
Satisfactory: Accurate performance with occassional supervision and clarification needed.
Unsatisfactory: Frequent inaccuracies in performance and frequent clarification needed.

	Superior	Satisfactory	Unsatisfactory
CLINICAL ASSESSMENT SKILLS			
1. Interviews (family of the elder who has Alzheimer's disease) about personality changes, irritability, forgetfulness, inattentiveness, judgement, signs of depression, and so on. Gains their perspective on how well the family is coping.			
2. Asks questions which give clues about confusion, including questions to gain evidence as to whether changes in mental status are acute or chronic onset (that is reversible or nonreversible).			
3. Reviews current mental status and mood; asks questions about recent and remote memory such as what was eaten for breakfast, name of grandmother; administers the Geriatric Depression Scale if appropriate.			
4. Reviews medications (especially those which are likely to cause sodium loss such as diuretics), use of sleeping pills and tranquilizers, other medications which contribute to confusion.			
5. Evaluates ability to do self care.			

6. Obtains history about falls, wandering away behaviour, continence, aggressive and assaultive behaviours, safety in the home such as use of the stove.			
Comments:			
DEVELOPING THE PLAN OF CARE			
1. Assessment data gained in the clinical assessment is comprehensive.			
2. Makes correct nursing diagnoses for actual or potential problems.			
3. Writes goals which are realistic, measurable and written in terms of the older person's accomplishment.			
4. Develops creative nursing interventions for all nursing diagnoses/problems.			
5. Describes the priority of all nursing diagnoses/problems.			
6. Care plans include safety, health promotion and education of the older person.			
Comments:			

General comments and recommendations:

STUDENT EVALUATION TOOLS

Assessment of Practical Skills

Module 10 - Mental health and aging

Student's Name: ____________________ Instructor's Name ____________________

Date of Clinical Experience: ____________________

Simulation Exercise: ____________________

Healthcare Setting: ____________________

EVALUATE THE STUDENT'S PERFORMANCE BY SCORING EACH ITEM USING THE FOLLOWING CRITERIA:

Superior: Accurate performance with minimal supervision and clarification needed.
Satisfactory: Accurate performance with occassional supervision and clarification needed.
Unsatisfactory: Frequent inaccuracies in performance and frequent clarification needed.

	Superior	Satisfactory	Unsatisfactory
CLINICAL ASSESSMENT SKILLS			
1. Uses advanced knowledge to identify biopsychosocial, cultural, educational and mental health care needs of selected clients and their families.			
2. Uses mental health assessment techniques in determining normals and deviations from clinical norms.			
3. Applies advanced knowledge to propose solutions to mental health care needs of selected clients, including wellness and self-care strategies.			
4. Demonstrates group strategies frequently used to maintain and/or restore the emotional well-being of older persons.			
Comments:			

DEVELOPING THE PLAN OF CARE			
1. Assessment data gained in the clinical assessment is comprehensive.			
2. Makes correct nursing diagnoses for actual or potential problems.			
3. Writes goals which are realistic, measurable and written in terms of the older person's accomplishment.			
4. Develops creative nursing interventions for all nursing diagnoses/problems.			
5. Describes the priority of all nursing diagnoses/problems.			
6. Care plans include safety, health promotion and education of the older person.			
Comments:			

General comments and recommendations:

STUDENT EVALUATION TOOLS

Assessment of Practical Skills

Module 11 - Supporting families in caregiving

Student's Name: ______________________ Instructor's Name ____________________

Date of Clinical Experience: ____

Simulation Exercise: ____

Healthcare Setting: ____

EVALUATE THE STUDENT'S PERFORMANCE BY SCORING EACH ITEM USING THE FOLLOWING CRITERIA:

Superior: Accurate performance with minimal supervision and clarification needed.
Satisfactory: Accurate performance with occassional supervision and clarification needed.
Unsatisfactory: Frequent inaccuracies in performance and frequent clarification needed.

	Superior	**Satisfactory**	**Unsatisfactory**
CLINICAL ASSESSMENT SKILLS			
1. Indicates knowledge of caregiver burden concepts and includes planning for relief from caregiver burden.			
2. Uses appropriate questions/methods to assess mistreatment and neglect to examine the older person.			
3. Incorporates knowledge of caregiver/public health/environment issues into planning care for the older person.			
4. Involves client in clinical, problem-identification and -solving process and encourages ways for the older person to be more independent.			
Comments:			

DEVELOPING THE PLAN OF CARE			
1. Assessment data gained in the clinical assessment is comprehensive.			
2. Makes correct nursing diagnoses for actual or potential problems.			
3. Writes goals which are realistic, measurable and written in terms of the older person's accomplishment.			
4. Develops creative nursing interventions for all nursing diagnoses/problems.			
5. Describes the priority of all nursing diagnoses/problems.			
6. Care plans include safety, health promotion and education of the older person.			
Comments:			

General comments and recommendations:

STUDENT EVALUATION TOOLS

Assessment of Practical Skills

Module 12 - Health promotion summary

Student's Name: ______________________ Instructor's Name ____________________

Date of Clinical Experience: ______________________________________

Simulation Exercise: ____

Healthcare Setting: ____

EVALUATE THE STUDENT'S PERFORMANCE BY SCORING EACH ITEM USING THE FOLLOWING CRITERIA:

Superior: Accurate performance with minimal supervision and clarification needed.
Satisfactory: Accurate performance with occassional supervision and clarification needed.
Unsatisfactory: Frequent inaccuracies in performance and frequent clarification needed.

	Superior	**Satisfactory**	**Unsatisfactory**
CLINICAL ASSESSMENT SKILLS			
1. Takes history of health risk behaviours such as smoking, alcohol use, salt and fat use, roughage in the diet, laxative use, falls and so on and provides appropriate counselling.			
2. Takes a sleep history including assessment of such factors as daytime sleepiness and napping, how sleep differs from previous patterns, whether sleep problems interfere with daily functioning, what measures are taken to help sleep, use of sleeping pills, exercise patterns, anxiety/stress.			
3. Conducts a nutritional assessment; uses the Nutrition Screen Levels I and II if helpful and appropriate; includes all aspects of dietary patterns such as ability to chew.			
4. Screens and performs necessary tests for hypertension, breast cancer, cervical cancer, colorectal cancer, and prostatic cancer.			
5. Interviews about immunization for *tetanus toxoid* and *hepatitis B*.			

6. Reviews medications, assesses for side effects, assesses for understanding of dose and purpose, instructs as necessary, and collaborates with other disciplines and/or refers as necessary.			
Comments:			
DEVELOPING THE PLAN OF CARE			
1. Assessment data gained in the clinical assessment is comprehensive.			
2. Makes correct nursing diagnoses for actual or potential problems.			
3. Writes goals which are realistic, measurable and written in terms of the older person's accomplishment.			
4. Develops creative nursing interventions for all nursing diagnoses/problems.			
5. Describes the priority of all nursing diagnoses/problems.			
6. Care plans include safety, health promotion and education of the older person.			
Comments:			

General comments and recommendations:

STUDENT EVALUATION TOOLS

Examination Questions

(Answer key on Annex1.46)

MODULE 1 - OVERVIEW

1. Which one of the following will **NOT** help older persons stay healthy and independent:

   a. understand age-related changes
   b. maximize the capabilities of older persons
   c. help them to take it easy
   d. instruct them in healthy lifestyles

2. Theories proposed to explain aging are organized as:

   a. fully explanatory and partially explanatory
   b. complete and incomplete
   c. genetic, biochemical and sociopsychological
   d. known and unknown

3. It is important to learn more about the health care of the elderly because:

   a. they are becoming a large segment of the population
   b. they are demanding their rights
   c. they are more important than younger age groups
   d. it is in fashion

4. Which of the following does **NOT** encourage quality health care for the elderly:

   a. promoting health and minimizing limitations
   b. maintaining independent lifestyles in their communities
   c. supporting family members in their efforts to sustain the well-being of their relatives
   d. keeping them away from distractions

5. Stereotypes about older persons usually come about because of:

   a. absence of factual information
   b. absence of good looks
   c. absence of good taste
   d. absence of money

6. Stereotyping:

   a. can be ignored
   b. can limit the potential of elderly persons
   c. is the scientific name for feeling old
   d. is an old fashioned idea

7. In the WEAR and TEAR theory of aging, continued use of the body is supposed to lead to worn out parts, similar to the breakdown and wearing out of old machinery. This could **NOT** explain aging because:

   a. continued use has little effect
   b. nothing ever wears out completely
   c. the human body can't be compared to machinery
   d. greater use leads to improvement in some systems such as muscles

8. The SOMATIC MUTATION THEORY states that low doses of radiation accelerate aging. The theory has been criticized for three reasons. Which of the following is NOT one of the reasons why this theory explains little about the aging process:

   a. sunscreens are now available to block out the harmful ultraviolet rays
   b. the effect of the sun occurs mainly in dividing cells while the effects of aging are seen mainly in cells that no longer divide
   c. the number of cells that undergo mutation is too small to account for overall aging
   d. most cells contain mechanisms for the repair of **DNA**

9. Which of the following theories explains that the critical factor in framing old age concerns is how well persons function in regard to <u>activities of daily living</u>?

   a. the functional capacity theory
   b. the activity theory
   c. the disengagement theory
   d. the personal meaning theory

10. The view that older people **WITHDRAW** from society is:

    a. the "adios" theory
    b. the disengagement theory
    c. the parting theory
    d. the absence theory

STUDENT EVALUATION TOOLS

Examination Questions

(Answer key on Annex1.46)

MODULE 2 (THE SENSES)

1. A friend tells you that she has "liver spots". The correct medical term for this is:

   a. brown spots
   b. age spots
   c. lentigo senilis
   d. missa luba

2. As one ages there are changes in the nerve fibres which affect the sense of smell. Which of the following is an important implication of change in smell?

   a. older people can no longer smell the roses
   b. older people no longer need to use perfumes
   c. older people might not smell smoke or spoiled food
   d. older people breathe through their mouths more

3. Which of the following colours do older people see BEST?

   a. blue, green, and purple
   b. red, yellow, and orange
   c. pink and blue
   d. black and white

4. Which of the following things in the environment can cause the greatest safety hazard to older persons?

   a. partially made beds
   b. partially swept floors
   c. partially opened doors
   d. partially clean dishes

5. The high frequency hearing loss typical in older persons is:

   a. presdonia
   b. presbycusis
   c. prestosterone
   d. prescontina

6. The greatest impact on the physical aging process overall and which is found in the loose connective tissue is from:

   a. collagen alone
   b. elastin alone
   c. both collagen and elastin
   d. colloids and proteins

7. All of the following could be clues that the older person is having trouble with hearing. Which response is **NOT** a sign of hearing impairment:

   a. withdrawing from conversation in groups
   b. giving a seemingly confused response to questions
   c. asking to have things repeated
   d. giving a correct answer to a direct question

8. The circle which forms around the iris in the eyes of older people and which is termed ARCUS SENILIS:

   a. needs to be corrected with surgery
   b. needs to be corrected with glasses
   c. is a normal age-related change
   d. should be corrected with laser beam

9. A frequent indication that older persons' taste buds are not functioning well is:

   a. they have a white coating on the tongue
   b. they add many spoonsful of sugar to their tea or coffee
   c. they have more saliva
   d. they pretend that they are dieting

10. A common **PROBLEM** (and not a normal age-related change) in vision is:

   a. greater sensitivity to glare
   b. formation of diabetic retinopathy
   c. greater difficulty reading with small print
   d. change in depth perception

STUDENT EVALUATION TOOLS

Examination Questions

(Answer key on Annex1.47)

MODULE 3 (THE MUSCULOSKELETAL SYSTEM)

1. Which of the following behaviours contribute to osteoporosis:

   a. smoking, alcohol, and lack of exercise
   b. physical activity, dancing, and swimming
   c. drinking tea, deep breathing, and losing weight
   d. knee bends, shopping, and weight lifting

2. As people get older, they lose height (become shorter). This is due to:

   a. the fact that they don't stand up straight
   b. the rest of the population has grown taller
   c. loss of bone mass in the vertebral discs
   d. inaccurate measurement

3. As one ages, muscle mass (that is muscle size):

   a. decreases
   b. increases
   c. stays about the same
   d. can go either way

4. As a result of changes in long bones and the spinal column, the gait of older people:

   a. becomes like a dancer
   b. is less stable and balanced when walking
   c. is more steady
   d. hardly changes at all

5. Changes in the bone of older people make which of the following a major danger?

   a. infection
   b. contagion
   c. allergy
   d. fractures

6. Changes in the the elasticity of chest and respiratory muscles mean that the lungs of older people have:

   a. smaller expansion
   b. larger expansion
   c. no expansion
   d. no change in expansion

7. Less muscle means less storage of glycogen (fuel for body energy). One implication of this is:

   a. older people need more calories
   b. older people should eat more sugar
   c. older people should stay close to restaurants
   d. older people have slower reactions to crisis or emergency situations

8. Osteoarthritis is:

   a. a normal age-related change
   b. an inflammatory disease frequent among older persons
   c. nearly the same as rheumatoid arthritis
   d. a rare occurrence

9. By 75 years of age, over 50% of older adults have which of the following diseases:

   a. tonsillitis
   b. cholecystitis
   c. osteoarthritis
   d. appendicitis

10. In helping older people who have problems with their joints and bones, one of the best things you can do to help them is:

   a. to anticipate their ADL needs and plan for them
   b. tell them to try harder
   c. do everything for them so that you feel better about their situation
   d. keep the joints immobile by using splints

STUDENT EVALUATION TOOLS

Examination Questions

(Answer key on Annex1.47)

MODULE 4 - URINARY SYSTEM

1. The glomerular filtration decreases nearly 50% between 20 and 90 years of age. This affects medications by:

   a. making them less potent, thereby diluting the effect
   b. not excreting them as quickly, often causing toxic effects
   c. forming stones which interfere with the effect
   d. causing no clinical problem in terms of effect

2. Older women who have urinary incontinence problems tend to have leakage or dribbling of urine. On the other hand, men who have urinary incontinence usually have retention with OVERFLOW. This is typically caused by:

   a. enlarged gall bladder
   b. enlarged liver
   c. enlarged prostate
   d. enlarged colon

3. The increase in glomerular filtration rate plus the smaller amount that the older person's bladder can hold do which of the following:

   a. cause older people to talk about their kidneys a lot
   b. cause older people to sleep later
   c. cause older people to measure their urine
   d. cause older people to get up frequently during the night to urinate

4. The antidiuretic hormone (ADH) works less effectively as one gets older, causing loss of sodium and fluid. A frequent sign of both hyponatremia and dehydration is:

   a. hunger
   b. confusion
   c. pink colour
   d. hysteria

5. People who have stress incontinence leak urine when they cough, laugh or sneeze. For this reason, they are **NOT GENERALLY** incontinent during the night. In discussing night-time continence with them, one other factor is important to mention as a cause of night-time incontinence. That is:

   a. rolling over in bed
   b. sitting up in bed
   c. lying on their backs in bed
   d. sexual activity in bed

6. The type of exercise recommended to help women control urinary incontinence is:

   a. aerobic
   b. high impact
   c. low impact
   d. kegel

7. Women who have had many children are likely to have more problems with urinary incontinence in later life.

   a. true
   b. false

8. An important consideration in working with families and older persons on the subject of incontinence is:

   a. control of appetite
   b. control of sleeping
   c. control of odours
   d. control of flatus

9. In older persons who have problems with incontinence, skin care is a major concern.

   a. true
   b. false

10. One of the dangers for elders who must get up at night to urinate is:

   a. the risk of not getting back to sleep
   b. the risk of getting a hunger attack while up
   c. the risk of getting a headache
   d. the risk of falling in the dark

STUDENT EVALUATION TOOLS

Examination Questions

(Answer key on Annex 1.48)

MODULE 5 - THE GASTROINTESTINAL SYSTEM

1. Cancer of the rectum is more common:

   a. in women
   b. in men
   c. in younger people
   d. with long term medication use

2. Which of the following should be encouraged to decrease the risk of constipation in older persons:

   a. good fluid intake and regular exercise
   b. limited fluid intake and regular exercise
   c. use of daily laxatives
   d. a soft or liquid diet

3. Many factors contribute to constipation in elderly persons and one of the most common ones is:

   a. fruit
   b. vegetables
   c. the side effects of medications
   d. meats and fish

4. As one gets older, (1) peristalsis decreases in the esophagus, (2) the stomach is slower in emptying and (3) less saliva is secreted. This can cause:

   a. crying
   b. choking
   c. biting
   d. chafing

5. Constipation in the elderly is **NOT** a normal age-related change

   a. true
   b. false

6. Hiatal hernia is **NOT** a normal age-related change

   a. true
   b. false

7. Because cancer of the colon and rectum increase with age, screens for occult (hidden) blood should be done routinely.

   a. true
   b. false

8. One approach to helping older persons with the problem of hiatal hernia is:

   a. to give small, frequent feedings of a bland diet
   b. to give large feedings of a bland diet
   c. to leave a diet alone
   d. to change to a completely liquid diet

9. Other types of cancer (besides colon and recturm) which increase with age (in the GI system) include:

   a. cancer of lips and jaw
   b. cancer of the mouth, stomach and liver
   c. cancer of the liver and spleen
   d. cancer of the stomach and spleen

10. Lack of privacy:

   a. rarely is a problem for older adults
   b. is just a fact of life
   c. can cause older persons to ignore the urge to defecate
   d. is a social problem

STUDENT EVALUATION TOOLS

Examination Questions

(Answer key on Annex 1.48)

MODULE 6 - CARDIOVASCULAR AND RESPIRATORY SYSTEMS

1. There are changes in the heart with age, but most of these have little functional significance. However, there is one thing which the heart does less well. That is:

   a. fall in love
   b. stay in love
   c. respond to stress or challenges
   d. flutter

2. Changes in the cardiovascular system make older persons more susceptible to fainting as a result of:

   a. orthostatic hypotension
   b. weak knees
   c. weak muscles
   d. cramps

3. Even if lifelong health habits have not been positive, beginning good health practices later in life can make a difference.

   a. true
   b. false

4. Decreased elasticity in lung tissue and muscles, and in the action of cilia, contribute to older people getting pneumonia more often than younger persons.

   a. true
   b. false

5. Which of the following is **NOT** recommended for helping to prevent strokes:

   a. lowering fat and salt in the diet
   b. increasing exercise
   c. eating a high fat/high cholesterol diet
   d. quitting smoking

6. Due to age-related changes in the lungs:

   a. the depth of the maximum breath which one can take becomes larger
   b. the depth of the maximum breath which one can take becomes smaller
   c. the sound of breathing is more labored
   d. the inhaled breath is different from the exhaled breath

7. In addition to pneumonia, another frequent infection of the respiratory system of older adults is:

   a. chronic obstructive lung disease
   b. asthma
   c. cancer
   d. tuberculosis

STUDENT EVALUATION TOOLS

Examination Questions

(Answer key on Annex 1.48)

MODULE 7 - AGE-RELATED CHANGES IN REPRODUCTIVE SYSTEMS AND LATE LIFE SEXUALITY

1. Menopause is considered complete when:

   a. hot flashes cease
   b. emotional stability ends
   c. a woman has been without periods for a year
   d. irritability goes away

2. Hormonal decline in women causes:

   a. increased risk for atherosclerotic plaques
   b. decreased risk for atherosclerotic plaques
   c. no change in risk for atherosclerotic plaques

3. Benefits of hormone replacement therapy (HRT) include:

   a. protection against constipation
   b. protection agains osteoporosis and elimination of the unpleasant symptoms of menopause
   c. protection against the flu
   d. protection against fever

4. Which of the following is **NOT** a known risk of hormone replacement therapy:

   a. formation of blood clots and hypertension
   b. development of noncancerous fibroid tumors in the uterus
   c. breast and endometrial cancers
   d. lung cancer

5. The expression of sexuality is affected by cultural forms.

   a. true
   b. false

6. Because the PH of the vagina becomes more alkaline with age, this predisposes older women to more:

   a. infertility
   b. menstruation
   c. infections
   d. pregnancies

7. Past 65 years of age, nearly all men have enlargement of the prostate.

   a. true
   b. false

8. As people get older, sexuality:

   a. decreases greatly
   b. remains an important part of the life experience
   c. becomes a thing of the past
   d. is no longer of concern to them

9. In counselling older persons about sexuality, recommendations should:

   a. not be too specific
   b. not be too lengthy
   c. not be included in discussions about other health problems
   d. not put them in conflict with their cultural or religious values

10. Alcohol and the side effects of medications can cause (older) men to have difficulty with erections.

   a. true
   b. false

STUDENT EVALUATION TOOLS

Examination Questions

(Answer key on Annex 1.49)

MODULE 8 - ENDOCRINE AND IMMUNE FUNCTION

1. As one gets older, the basil metabolic rate (BMR) goes down but it is still adequate for normal functioning of older adults.

   a. true
   b. false

2. Although inconclusive, there is evidence that in older persons, the immune function:

   a. increases
   b. decreases
   c. stays the same
   d. changes from time to time

3. Older people are no more likely to get non-insulin dependent diabetes mellitus (NIDDM) than younger people.

   a. true
   b. false

4. In older people, diabetes is often found by chance during the search for the cause of other problems such as:

   a. visual disturbance and delayed healing
   b. measles and excessive hair growth
   c. baldness
   d. flu symptoms

5. Two of the greatest problems associated with diabetes are:

   a. lack of money and difficulty driving
   b. back aches and stomach pains
   c. salt and pepper intolerance
   d. infection of feet and legs, and visual problems

6. Support for a reduced immune response in older adults is demonstrated by the increased tendency for:

   a. liver disease
   b. thyroid problems
   c. pneumonia and cancer
   d. osteoporosis

STUDENT EVALUATION TOOLS

Examination Questions

(Answer key on Annex 1.49)

MODULE 9 - DEMENTING ILLNESS AND CHANGES IN THE BRAIN

1. As one gets older, there is a loss of brain cells. The significance of this is:

   a. a cell transplant is indicated
   b. the lost cells will regenerate on their own
   c. the remaining cells are more than enough for learning and remembering
   d. the significance is not known

2. ACUTE dementia is due to causes which can be reversed. A frequent cause of this type of dementia is:

   a. cerebrovascular accident
   b. Alzheimer's disease
   c. multiple infarcts
   d. electrolyte imbalance, especially hyponatremia (loss of sodium)

3. In CHRONIC or nonreversible dementia the course is one of gradual but inevitable decline.

   a. true
   b. false

4. The brains of persons with Alzheimer's disease are characterized by the presence of:

   a. fatty deposits
   b. senile plaques and neurofibrillary tangles
   c. calcium deposits
   d. lack of gray matter

5. There is evidence that the chromosome responsible for <u>late onset</u> Alzheimer's disease (which is typical in old age) is on chromosome number:

   a. 21 - the same one as for Down's syndrome
   b. 19

6. Which of the following could be a symptom of early stages of Alzheimer's disease:

   a. wearing a white shoe on one foot and a blue shoe on the other
   b. singing the words along with a tune
   c. paying bills promptly
   d. laughing at a good joke

7. Which of the following become frequent management problems as dementing illness progresses:

    a. incontinence and wandering away
    b. headaches and wandering away
    c. stomach cramps and wandering away
    d. double vision and wandering away

8. One of the main things to remember about helping families take care of their older relatives who have dementia, is that they need arrangements for periodic relief of their responsibilities. This is done:

    a. so that they do not become excited and get the flu
    b. so that they do not become exhausted and have fits of laughter
    c. so that they do not become exhausted and socially isolated
    d. so that they do not become excited and go dancing

9. Reality orientation should be done:

    a. only in groups
    b. only one-to-one (individually) while the demented elderly person is awake
    c. both in groups and one-to-one (individually) while the demented elderly person is awake
    d. however the health care worker decides

10. Which of the following things can cause agitated behaviour in older persons who are demented:

    a. smiling at the person
    b. reducing the amount of stimulation
    c. being gentie
    d. trying to force them

STUDENT EVALUATION TOOLS

Examination Questions

(Answer key on Annex 1.50)

MODULE 10 - MENTAL HEALTH AND AGING

1. Older adults and their families may deny the existence of mental health problems. Of the reasons which follow, which one does NOT explain their denial:

   a. they feel these problems are shameful
   b. they think suffering should be endured
   c. they want to appear in control to maintain their dignity
   d. they are too busy to get help

2. A positive mental outlook is essential to healthy aging.

   a. true
   b. false

3. Group work with old-age groups requires some special skills. Which of the following is typically NOT provided by group leaders in these groups:

   a. emotional support and encouragement
   b. analysis of personality problems
   c. focus on problem-solving
   d. help to discover sources of hope and motivation

4. Which of the following describes a reminiscence group:

   a. it is part of a normal life review process
   b. it is not done by very many older people
   c. the focus is on making one feel productive
   d. it is especially effective with demented elderly persons

5. The most common mental health problem among older adults is:

   a. paranoia
   b. schizophrenia
   c. mania
   d. depression

6. Many things contribute to depression in older persons. Which of the following does **NOT** usually contribute to depression:

    a. death of loved ones
    b. chronic illness and pain
    c. lack of control
    d. stimulating activities

7. In older people, depression may not present as the usual picture of sadness. Instead it may:

    a. look like dementia OR agitation
    b. look like it will go away on its own
    c. look like nothing to worry about
    d. look like one would expect in old age

8. In groups which are held to help older adults deal with grief over the death of loved one, the discussion centres around:

    a. repeating the mourning many times
    b. expressing regret about the lost time
    c. expressing sadness but talking about the importance of the relationship and the wonderful memories
    d. fears of their own death

9. The goals for groups which are conducted to support families most often are to:

    a. educate them about the aging process or illness of the elderly person, gain cooperation in the plan of care for the elderly person, and reduce anxiety and burden
    b. avoid conflict with them later on in the plan of care and avoid surprises

10. In promoting the mental health and well being of older adults, one of the most important things to do is:

    a. make them feel grateful
    b. tell them they are one in a million
    c. find areas where they can have a sense of control
    d. tell them to think about flowers

STUDENT EVALUATION TOOLS

Examination Questions

(Answer key on Annex 1.50)

MODULE 11 - SUPPORTING FAMILES IN CAREGIVING

1. All people are living longer and this has increased the number of generations living together. In addition to the problem of lack of space, another concern that this can cause is lack of:

   a. clean air
   b. privacy

2. When older persons are sick, health care workers often concentrate on the needs of the elderly person, and ignore the needs of the caregiver. In this situation, the caregiver is called:

   a. the second class citizen
   b. the silent partner
   c. the hidden patient
   d. the complainer

3. Caregiver burden is:

   a. a myth
   b. the physical, emotional, social and financial costs associated with the caregiving experience
   c. something heavy they must lift
   d. the weight of the caregiver

4. Assessinig the degree of caregiver burden is difficult because:

   a. it has large and small factors
   b. it has old and new factors
   c. it is both an objective and subjective experience
   d. it is socially unacceptable

5. Caregivers typically experience much:

   a. stress
   b. hopefulness
   c. laughter
   d. sweetness

6. The idea of <u>induced dependency</u> is that:

   a. caregivers become dependent themselves
   b. caregivers avoid becoming dependent themselves
   c. caregivers make health care workers dependent
   d. caregivers can help elderly persons with self-care beyond that required, thereby reducing the elderly persons' ability to care for themselves

7. Induced dependency done by caregivers often occurs unintentionally because it is:

   a. faster to do the care than to let the elderly person do it
   b. more accurate to do the care than to let the elderly person do it

8. The two <u>types</u> of elder abuse which can occur are:

   a. one time and multiple time
   b. past and present
   c. mistreatment or neglect

9. Abuse can be further divided into:

   a. old and new
   b. settings
   c. physical and psychological

10. A very important part of supporting famiies in their caregiving is:

    a. keeping them out of the workforce
    b. coordinating needed resources in the community
    c. preparing meals for them

STUDENT EVALUATION TOOLS

Examination Questions

(Answer key on Annex 1.51)

MODULE 12 - HEALTH PROMOTION SUMMARY

1. Which of the following are needs for health promotion of older adults:

   a. education about drugs, diet, safety and exercise
   b. immunizations
   c. screening for cancer, diabetes, and hypertension
   d. all of the above

2. Which of the following immunizations are recommended for older persons:

   a. flu and polio
   b. tetanus toxoid and hepatitis B
   c. tetanus toxoid and polio
   d. malaria and polio

3. Although nutritional requirements are essentially the same for older and younger adults, there are a few differences. One of them is that:

   a. younger people require more tea
   b. older people need less calories
   c. older people need to diet more
   d. younger people need to diet more

4. The risk and incidence of cancer of the breast DECREASE with age.

   a. true
   b. false

5. The risk and incidence of cancer of the prostate INCREASE with age.

   a. true
   b. false

6. Because of normal age-related changes in the liver, kidneys, muscle mass and total body fluid, older people have which reaction to alcohol:

   a. they need larger amounts to get intoxicated
   b. there is no particular reaction one way or the other
   c. they get intoxicated with smaller amounts
   d. they sweat it out

7. Which of the following is <u>true</u> about the sleep of older people:

    a. their sleep patterns are unchanged
    b. they spend less time in all four stages of sleep
    c. they dream constantly instead of sleeping
    d. they do not dream in colour

8. Most of the following can interfere with sleep in older people. Which one **DOES NOT** <u>interfere</u> with sleep but promotes it:

    a. fear, anxiety and worry
    b. chronic pair or the side effects of certain medications
    c. loss of sleeping partner
    d. a backrub

9. In trying to overcome problems with sleep in older people, which of the following should be ENCOURAGED:

    a. weigthlifting, backbends and some television
    b. warm milk, regular exercise well before bedtime and avoidance of sleeping pills
    c. sleeping pills and exercise immediately before bed
    d. cold milk, a movie and concentration

10. The main concern about preventing accidents in older people is that:

    a. accidents can be expensive to treat
    b. they lead to immobility and loss of function
    c. they hurt a lot
    d. they look terrible

STUDENT EVALUATION TOOLS

Answer Key

MODULE 1 - OVERVIEW

1. (c) help them to take it easy
2. (c) genetic, biochemical and sociopsychological
3. (a) they are becoming a large segment of the population
4. (d) keeping them away from distractions
5. (a) absence of factual information
6. (b) can limit the potential of elderly persons
7. (d) greater use leads to improvement in some systems such as muscles
8. (a) sunscreens are now available to block out the harmful effects of ultraviolet rays
9. (a) functional capacity theory
10. (b) the disengagement theory

MODULE 2 (THE SENSES)

1. (c) lentigo senilis
2. (c) older people might not smell smoke or spoiled food
3. (b) red, yellow, and orange
4. (c) partially-opened doors
5. (b) presbycusis
6. (c) collagen and elastin
7. (d) giving a correct answer to a direct question
8. (c) is a normal age-related change
9. (b) they add many spoonsful of sugar to their coffee
10. (b) formation of diabetic retinopathy

MODULE 3 (THE MUSCULOSKELETAL SYSTEM)

1. (a) smoking, alcohol use and lack of exercise
2. (c) loss of bone mass in the vertebral discs
3. (a) decreases
4. (b) is less stable and balanced when walking
5. (d) fractures
6. (a) smaller expansion
7. (d) older people have slower reactions to crisis or emergency
8. (b) an inflammatory disease frequent among older persons
9. (c) osteoarthritis
10. (a) to anticipate their ADL needs and plan for them

MODULE 4 - THE URINARY SYSTEM

1. (b) not excreting them as quickly, often causing toxic effects
2. (c) enlarged prostate
3. (d) cause older people to get up frequently during the night to urinate
4. (b) confusion
5. (d) sexual activity in bed
6. (d) kegel
7. (a) true
8. (c) control of odours
9. (a) true
10. (d) the risk of falling in the dark

MODULE 5 - THE GASTROINTESTINAL SYSTEM

1. (b) in men
2. (a) good fluid intake and regular exercise
3. (c) the side effects of medications
4. (b) choking
5. (a) true
6. (a) true
7. (a) true
8. (a) to give small, frequent feedings of a bland diet
9. (b) cancer of the mouth, stomach and liver
10. (c) can cause older persons to ignore the urge to defecate

MODULE 6 - CARDIOVASCULAR AND RESPIRATORY SYSTEMS

1. (c) respond to stress or challenges
2. (a) orthostatic hypotension
3. (a) true
4. (a) true
5. (c) eating a high fat/high cholesterol diet
6. (b) the depth of the maximum breath which one can take becomes smaller
7. (d) tuberculosis

MODULE 7 - AGE-RELATED CHANGES IN THE REPRODUCTIVE SYSTEM AND LATE LIFE SEXUALITY

1. (a) a woman has been without periods for a year
2. (a) increased risk for atherosclerotic plaques
3. (b) protection against osteoporosis and the unpleasant symptoms of menopause
4. (d) cancer of the lung
5. (a) true

6. (c) infections

7. (a) true

8. (b) remains an important part of the life experience

9. (d) should not put them in conflict with their cultural or religious values

10. (a) true

MODULE 8 - ENDOCRINE AND IMMUNE FUNCTION

1. (a) true

2. (b) decreases

3. (a) true

4. (a) visual disturbance and delayed healing

5. (d) infection of feet and legs and visual problems

6. (c) pneumonia and cancer

MODULE 9 - DEMENTING ILLNESS AND CHANGES IN THE BRAIN

1. (c) the remaining cells are more than enough for learning and remembering

2. (d) electrolyte imbalance, especially hyponatremia (loss of sodium)

3. (a) true

4. (b) senile plaques and neurofibrillary tangles

5. (b) 19

6. (a) wearing a white shoe on one foot and a blue shoe on the other

7. (a) incontinence and wandering away

8. (c) so that they do not become exhausted and socially isolated

9. (c) both in groups and in one-to-one (individual) while the demented elderly person is awake

10. (d) trying to force them

MODULE 10 -MENTAL HEALTH AND AGING

1. (d) they are too busy to get help
2. (a) true
3. (b) analysis of personality problems
4. (a) it is part of a normal life review process
5. (d) depression
6. (d) stimulating activities
7. (a) look like dementia OR agitation
8. (c) expressing sadness but talking about the importance of the relationship and the wonderful memories
9. (a) educate them about the aging process or illness of the elderly person, gain cooperation in the plan of care for the elderly person, and reduce anxiety and burden
10. (c) find areas where they can have a sense of control

MODULE 11 -SUPPORTING FAMILIES IN CAREGIVING

1. (b) privacy
2. (c) the hidden patient
3. (b) the physical, emotional, social and financial costs associated with the caregiving experience
4. (c) it is both an objective and subjective experience
5. (a) stress
6. (d) caregivers can help elderly persons with self-care beyond that required, thereby the elderly person's ability to care for themselves
7. (a) faster to do the care than to let the elderly do it
8. (c) mistreatment or neglect
9. (c) physical and psychological
10. (b) coordinating needed resources in the community

MODULE 12 -HEALTH PROMOTION SUMMARY

1. (d) all of the above

2. (b) tetanus toxoid and hepatitis B

3. (b) older people need less calories

4. (b) false

5. (a) true

6. (c) they get intoxicated with smaller amounts

7. (b) they spend less time in all stages of sleep

8. (a) backrub

9. (b) warm milk, regular exercise well before bedtime and avoidance of sleeping pills

10. (b) they lead to immobility and loss of function

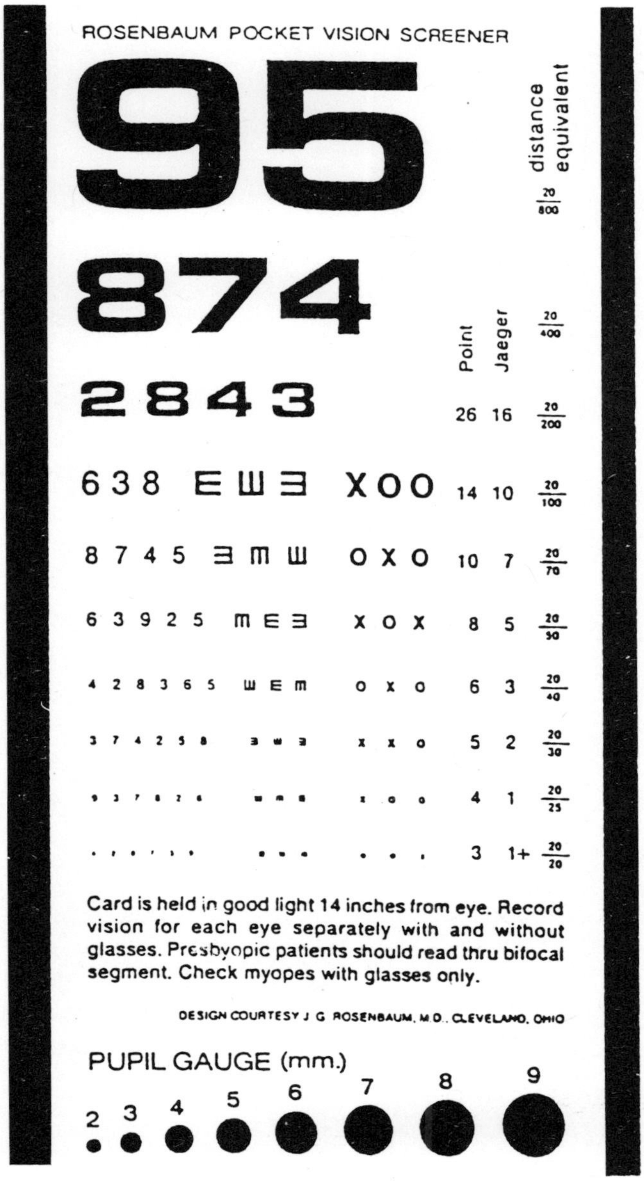
ROSENBAUM POCKET VISION SCREENER
95
distance equivalent
20/800
874
Point Jaeger 20/400
2843 26 16 20/200
638 EШ∃ XOO 14 10 20/100
8745 ∃ΠШ OXO 10 7 20/70
63925 ΠE∃ XOX 8 5 20/50
428365 ШEΠ OXO 6 3 20/40
5 2 20/30
4 1 20/25
3 1+ 20/20
Card is held in good light 14 inches from eye. Record vision for each eye separately with and without glasses. Presbyopic patients should read thru bifocal segment. Check myopes with glasses only.
DESIGN COURTESY J. G. ROSENBAUM, M.D., CLEVELAND, OHIO
PUPIL GAUGE (mm.)
2 3 4 5 6 7 8 9

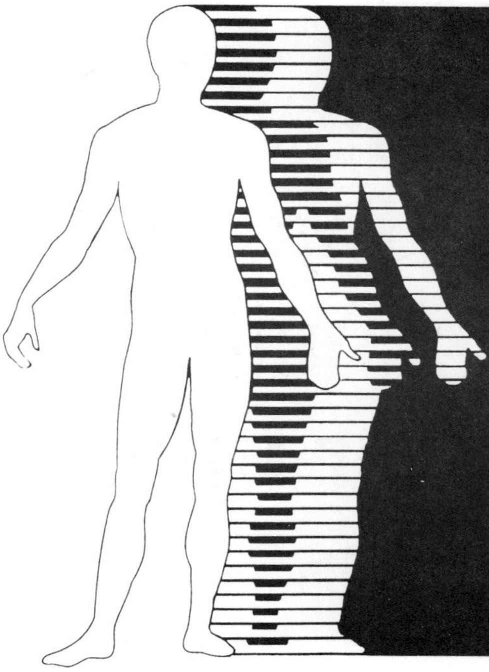

Nutrition Screening Manual for Professionals Caring for Older Americans

Nutrition Screening Initiative

A project of:

AMERICAN ACADEMY
OF FAMILY PHYSICIANS

THE AMERICAN
DIETETIC ASSOCIATION

NATIONAL COUNCIL
ON THE AGING, INC.

Nutrition Screening Manual for Professionals Caring for Older Americans

Nutrition Screening Initiative

A project of:

AMERICAN ACADEMY
OF FAMILY PHYSICIANS

THE AMERICAN
DIETETIC ASSOCIATION

NATIONAL COUNCIL
ON THE AGING, INC.

THE NUTRITION SCREENING INITIATIVE
2626 Pennsylvania Avenue, N.W., Suite 301, Washington, D.C. 20037 (202) 625-1662

The Nutrition Screening Initiative is made possible in part through a grant from Ross Laboratories, a division of Abbott Laboratories.

TABLE OF CONTENTS

Nutrition Screening Saves Time, Money, and Lives

Within this manual, you will find guidelines for administering three important tools designed to focus attention on the nutritional status of older Americans. While proper nutrition is critical to the good health of all Americans, older adults are at disproportionate risk for a number of reasons: difficulties in eating or swallowing, low income, adverse drug-nutrient interactions, alcohol abuse, depression, reduced appetite, functional disabilities, impaired taste and smell, and many others. In fact, over 85% of older adults suffer from chronic diseases that could benefit from dietary intervention. By taking a few extra minutes to screen for existing and potential problems, you will almost certainly save the older persons with whom you interact the time, expense, and discomfort of a future illness brought on or made worse by poor nutritional status and possibly even save their lives.

The checklist and screens are simple, brief, and clearly laid out to help you quickly identify individuals who may require nutrition counseling, social or health services, or medical and nutritional intervention. They are generic tools designed to encourage systematic evaluation of nutritional status. The tools will not be specifically appropriate to each and every health and social service setting in which they may be used. Rather, the tools' flexible design should allow a variety of professionals to adapt them to meet the needs of their clients or patients.

In addition to the checklist and screens, this manual includes guidelines for understanding the questions and clinical tests and for interpreting the results. Appropriate tables, figures, or laboratory values are provided for measures on the Level II Screen. However, the manual will not provide explicit instructions for each item on the checklist and screens; if you have additional questions about using the tools, you may want to contact the Nutrition Screening Initiative for information on training seminars and workshops in your area.

"DETERMINE Your Nutritional Health" Checklist

The "DETERMINE Your Nutritional Health" Checklist is a public awareness tool that can be self-administered or conducted by anyone who interacts with older family members, friends, or clients. The Checklist will help older Americans realize that they may be at increased risk for a nutritional problem, and a simple mnemonic DETERMINE will highlight the warning signs of poor nutritional status. For many people, becoming aware of the factors that affect their nutritional health will prompt them to improve their eating habits, modify their lifestyle, and, if necessary, seek professional help, thus reducing their risk of nutrition-related health problems.

Level I Screen

The Level I Screen offers a simple method for separating those individuals who should be referred for evaluation and possible intervention from those who would benefit from other medical or community services. This screen, which can be administered by professionals in health or social service programs, includes questions regarding height and weight, eating habits and lifestyle, and an assessment of socioeconomic and functional status. The Level I Screen will help to identify those individuals who may be candidates for home meal delivery, assistance with shopping or cooking, congregate meal programs, or nutrition therapy and education.

Level II Screen

For those older adults whose Checklist or Level I Screen indicates a potentially serious nutritional or medical problem, the Level II Screen provides some sensitive measurements that can be taken by a health care professional alone or as part of a complete physical examination. This screen includes more specific diagnostic information, such as a detailed history of weight change and laboratory and clinical indicators of protein calorie malnutrition, obesity, and other nutrition-related disorders. As with the Level I Screen, issues that can and should be addressed by specific health and social service professionals are clearly flagged to save time, money, and confusion.

For those of you who will be combining these screens with your organization's existing instruments, the Nutrition Screening Initiative would suggest that you take a moment to compare the information being collected and how you usually apply this information. For example, if you assess functional status or dietary intake to determine an individual's eligibility for home-delivered meals, you could take a fresh look at this information to check for increased risk of poor nutritional status. Clearly there is no need to duplicate data collection nor to create more paperwork for anyone. We would merely ask that you keep in mind the importance of reviewing the nutritional status of your clients or patients on a regular basis. You might also consider adding certain questions from the Level I Screen to your existing tools to ensure that the older adults with whom you work are getting the most out of your program by having their nutritional health monitored.

Definitions

Frequently, the definitions and standards used to document the occurrence, extent, causes, and remedies of poor nutritional status among older adults generate lively debate. The following definitions and standards summarize the multidisciplinary consensus reached at the conference, Nutrition Screening I: Toward a Common View.

Poor Nutritional Status includes not only deficiency, dehydration, undernutrition, nutritional imbalances, and obesity but other excesses such as alcohol abuse. In addition, inappropriate dietary intakes for conditions that have nutritional implications and the presence of an underlying physical or mental illness with treatable nutritional implications are included. Finally, it also encompasses evidence that nutritional status may be deteriorating over time. Such evidence may be derived from clear-cut objective clinical signs, by nonspecific clinical evidence, by responses to direct, specific questions about diet and nutrition (even if complaints are not volunteered), and by reliable reports from third parties (family, friends, caregivers, aides, social workers).

Risk Factors of poor nutritional status are characteristics that are associated with an increased likelihood of poor nutritional status. They include the presence of various acute or chronic disease diagnoses and conditions, inadequate quantity or quality of food (which suggests inappropriate food consumption), poverty, dependency, and medication use.

Indicators of poor nutritional status are generally quantitative and include specific food components in diets; dietary, clinical, anthropometric, hematologic, and other biochemical measurements related to specific food components; and health conditions or diseases that may be associated with them. Changes in these indicators over time is of particular importance. Major Indicators, which in general are quantifiable, if they are abnormal to a certain defined extext, mandate consideration of nutritional factors. Minor Indicators are less specific and/or quantifiable, and include some individual specific nutritional deficits.

Nutrition Screening is the process of discovering characteristics known to be associated with dietary or nutritional problems. Its purpose is to identify individuals who are at high risk of nutritional problems or who have poor nutritional status. Intervention is facilitated when screening is used.

The following are the risk factors as well as the major and minor indicators of poor nutritional status:

Risk Factors

Inappropriate food intake
Poverty
Social isolation
Dependency/disability
Acute/chronic diseases or conditions
Chronic medication use
Advanced age (80+)

Major Indicators

Weight loss
Under-/overweight
Low serum albumin
Change in functional status
Inappropriate food intake
Mid-arm muscle circumference
< 10th percentile
Triceps skinfold
< 10th percentile or >95th percentile
Obesity
Nutrition-related disorders
Osteoporosis
Osteomalacia
Folate deficiency
B12 deficiency

Minor Indicators

Alcoholism
Cognitive impairment
Chronic renal insufficiency
Multiple concurrent medications
Malabsorption syndromes
Anorexia, nausea. dysphagia
Change in bowel habit
Fatigue, apathy, memory loss
Poor oral /dental status, dehydration
Poorly healing wounds
Loss of subcutaneous fat and/or muscle mass
Fluid retention
Reduced iron, ascorbic acid, zinc

Overview

As with many public health campaigns, nutrition screening will be most effective when individual Americans take the initiative to monitor their own nutritional health. This tool describes in simple language a series of warning signs of poor nutritional status in older Americans, similar to the warning signs used to assist in the early detection of cancer. The goal is to raise consciousness about the importance of nutrition to an individual's health status.

The "DETERMINE Your Nutritional Health" Checklist consists of two elements: a self-assessment protocol that, through a series of statements, helps people recognize aspects of their eating habits and lifestyle that may place them at nutritional risk; and a mnemonic device (DETERMINE) designed to provide basic education on nutritional risk factors and indicators and to remind both the public and health professionals about the warning signs of poor nutritional health.

This tool has undergone considerable review and testing. Groups of older adults with varied ethnic, age, income, and educational backgrounds were asked to evaluate the usefulness, format, and credibility of the document. In addition, data collected by the National Center for Health Statistics, the New England Research Institute, and the Boston University School of Public Health were used as guides for the Checklist's wording, content, design, and scoring. This Checklist will be distributed across the United States as part of an aggressive campaign aimed at making the public aware of the potential nutritional problems in older Americans.

We hope that you will use the Checklist in your daily interactions with older patients and clients. When indicated, we hope that you will take appropriate action when you feel that it will benefit the older adult with whom you are working.

DETERMINE YOUR NUTRITIONAL HEALTH

The Warning Signs of poor nutritional health are often overlooked. Use this checklist to find out if you or someone you know is at nutritional risk.

Read the statements below. Circle the number in the yes column for those that apply to you or someone you know. For each yes answer, score the number in the box. Total your nutritional score.

	YES
I have an illness or condition that made me change the kind and/or amount of food I eat.	2
I eat fewer than 2 meals per day.	3
I eat few fruits or vegetables, or milk products.	2
I have 3 or more drinks of beer, liquor or wine almost every day.	2
I have tooth or mouth problems that make it hard for me to eat.	2
I don't always have enough money to buy the food I need.	4
I eat alone most of the time.	1
I take 3 or more different prescribed or over-the-counter drugs a day.	1
Without wanting to, I have lost or gained 10 pounds in the last 6 months.	2
I am not always physically able to shop, cook and/or feed myself.	2
TOTAL	

Total Your Nutritional Score. If it's —

0-2 **Good!** Recheck your nutritional score in 6 months.

3-5 **You are at moderate nutritional risk.** See what can be done to improve your eating habits and lifestyle. Your office on aging, senior nutrition program, senior citizens center or health department can help. Recheck your nutritional score in 3 months.

6 or more **You are at high nutritional risk.** Bring this checklist the next time you see your doctor, dietitian or other qualified health or social service professional. Talk with them about any problems you may have. Ask for help to improve your nutritional health.

These materials developed and distributed by the Nutrition Screening Initiative, a project of:

AMERICAN ACADEMY OF FAMILY PHYSICIANS

THE AMERICAN DIETETIC ASSOCIATION

NATIONAL COUNCIL ON THE AGING, INC.

Remember that warning signs suggest risk, but do not represent diagnosis of any condition. Turn the page to learn more about the Warning Signs of poor nutritional health.

The Nutrition Checklist is based on the Warning Signs described below. Use the word DETERMINE to remind you of the Warning Signs.

DISEASE

Any disease, illness or chronic condition which causes you to change the way you eat, or makes it hard for you to eat, puts your nutritional health at risk. Four out of five adults have chronic diseases that are affected by diet. Confusion or memory loss that keeps getting worse is estimated to affect one out of five or more of older adults. This can make it hard to remember what, when or if you've eaten. Feeling sad or depressed, which happens to about one in eight older adults, can cause big changes in appetite, digestion, energy level, weight and well-being.

EATING POORLY

Eating too little and eating too much both lead to poor health. Eating the same foods day after day or not eating fruit, vegetables, and milk products daily will also cause poor nutritional health. One in five adults skip meals daily. Only 13% of adults eat the minimum amount of fruit and vegetables needed. One in four older adults drink too much alcohol. Many health problems become worse if you drink more than one or two alcoholic beverages per day.

TOOTH LOSS/ MOUTH PAIN

A healthy mouth, teeth and gums are needed to eat. Missing, loose or rotten teeth or dentures which don't fit well or cause mouth sores make it hard to eat.

ECONOMIC HARDSHIP

As many as 40% of older Americans have incomes of less than $6,000 per year. Having less--or choosing to spend less--than $25-30 per week for food makes it very hard to get the foods you need to stay healthy.

REDUCED SOCIAL CONTACT

One-third of all older people live alone. Being with people daily has a positive effect on morale, well-being and eating.

MULTIPLE MEDICINES

Many older Americans must take medicines for health problems. Almost half of older Americans take multiple medicines daily. Growing old may change the way we respond to drugs. The more medicines you take, the greater the chance for side effects such as increased or decreased appetite, change in taste, constipation, weakness, drowsiness, diarrhea, nausea, and others. Vitamins or minerals when taken in large doses act like drugs and can cause harm. Alert your doctor to everything you take.

INVOLUNTARY WEIGHT LOSS/GAIN

Losing or gaining a lot of weight when you are not trying to do so is an important warning sign that must not be ignored. Being overweight or underweight also increases your chance of poor health.

NEEDS ASSISTANCE IN SELF CARE

Although most older people are able to eat, one of every five have trouble walking, shopping, buying and cooking food, especially as they get older.

ELDER YEARS ABOVE AGE 80

Most older people lead full and productive lives. But as age increases, risk of frailty and health problems increase. Checking your nutritional health regularly makes good sense.

The Nutrition Screening Initiative, 2626 Pennsylvania Avenue, NW, Suite 301, Washington, DC 20037

The Nutrition Screening Initiative is funded in part by a grant from Ross Laboratories, a division of Abbott Laboratories.

Overview

We all recognize that many older Americans are at high risk of nutritional deficits, excesses, and imbalances that may negatively affect their health and well-being. The goal of the Nutrition Screening Initiative is to identify persons who are at risk before their health has deteriorated to the point that they must be medicated, institutionalized, or hospitalized. This Level I Screen has been designed to single out those older adults who need medical or nutritional attention and, just as importantly, to help health and social service workers determine what preventive action can be taken to ensure that the majority of older Americans do not become malnourished. Early identification of problems and appropriate intervention increases the likelihood that older people will live longer, more fulfilling, and more productive lives.

Carefully selected screening questions have been divided among four sections that correspond to the four most common types of action to be taken in assisting older adults to eat a healthy diet. The first section on body weight and change in weight is perhaps the most important because it will alert you as to whether the individual who you are screening should see a physician immediately. The next area screened examines the person's actual eating habits. Positive responses to these statements should flag the need to see a dentist, dietitian, or alcohol abuse counselor. The focus then shifts to problems in socioeconomic and functional status that would best be solved by a case manager, home health care service, social worker, or financial assistance. You might want to jot down names and phone numbers of physicians (particularly those specializing in geriatric medicine), clinics, dietitians, dentists, psychologists, services, and agencies to have on hand when screening older adults.

Many of the questions on this screen are similar to those asked by home health care agencies and state-run community care programs. If you are familiar with this type of assessment, please rely on your prior training and experience when interpreting the responses that you receive from older adults. If you are a newcomer to this type of screening, take a conservative approach: if an individual gives you an ambiguous or vacillating response, assume they are at risk for that particular factor and place a check by the statement on the screen. Even if no serious problem currently exists, you will probably prevent the development of future problems, and a health care or social service professional will be able to determine what level of assistance is required to maintain or restore nutritional health.

If when you complete the Level I Screen it is apparent that the individual requires medical attention, you must determine whether the individual is able or willing to contact his or her own physician or whether an appointment should be made. If the individual indicates that he or she is willing to make an appointment, stress the importance of doing so soon. If the individual cannot or does not want to be responsible for scheduling a doctor's visit, then you or the person's case worker might want to assist them by scheduling an appointment.

Level I Screen

Body Weight

Measure height to the nearest inch or centimetre and weight to the nearest pound org. Record the values below and mark them on the Body Mass Index (BMI) scale to the right. Then use a straight edge (ruler) to connect the two points and circle the spot where this straight line crosses the center line (body mass index). Record the number below.

Healthy older adults should have a BMI between 24 and 27.

Height (in/cm):______________
Weight (lbs/kg):______________
Body Mass Index:______________
(number from center column)

Check any boxes that are true for the individual:

- ☐ Has lost or gained 10 pounds or 4.5 kg (or more) in the past 6 months.
- ☐ Body mass index <24
- ☐ Body mass index >27

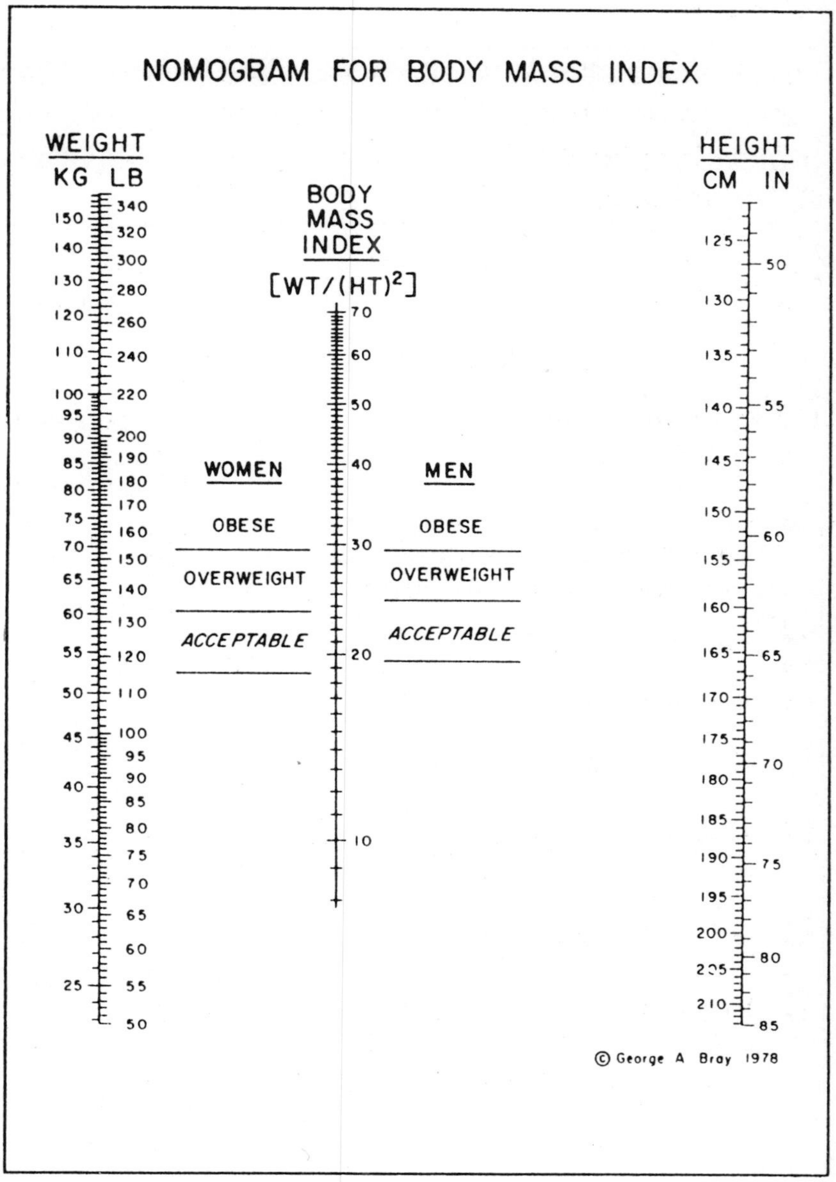

For the remaining sections, please ask the individual which of the statements (if any) is true for him or her and place a check by each that applies.

Eating Habits

- ☐ Does not have enough food to eat each day
- ☐ Usually eats alone
- ☐ Does not eat anything on one or more days each month
- ☐ Has poor appetite
- ☐ Is on a special diet
- ☐ Eats vegetables two or fewer times daily
- ☐ Eats milk or milk products once or not at all daily
- ☐ Eats fruit or drinks fruit juice once or not at all daily
- ☐ Eats breads, cereals, pasta, rice or other grains five or fewer times daily
- ☐ Has difficulty chewing or swallowing
- ☐ Has more than one alcoholic drink per day (if woman); more than two drinks per day (if man)
- ☐ Has pain in mouth, teeth, or gums

Name:

Date:

A physician should be contacted if the individual has gained or lost 10 pounds or 4.5 kg unexpectedly or without intending to during the past 6 months. A physician should also be notified if the individual's bodymass index is above 27 or below 24.

Living environment

(Please adapt to local conditions)

- ❑ Lives on an income of less than $6000 per year* (per individual in the household, or an appropriate figure for your country)
- ❑ Lives alone
- ❑ Is housebound
- ❑ Is concerned about home security
- ❑ Lives in a home with inadequate heating or cooling
- ❑ Does not have a stove and/or refrigerator
- ❑ Is unable or prefers not to spend enough money on food*

Functional Status

Usually or always needs assistance with (check each that apply)

- ❑ Bathing
- ❑ Dressing
- ❑ Grooming
- ❑ Toileting
- ❑ Eating
- ❑ Walking or moving about
- ❑ Travelling (outside the home)
- ❑ Preparing food
- ❑ Shopping for food or other necessities

If you have checked one or more statements on this screen, the individual you have interviewed may be at risk for poor nutritional status. Please refer this individual to the appropriate health care or social service professional in your area. For example, a dietician should be contacted for problems with selecting, preparing, or eating a healthy diet, or a dentist if the individual experiences pain or difficulty when chewing or swallowing. Those individuals whose income, lifestyle, or functional status may endanger their nutritional and overall health should be referred to available community services: home-delivered meals, congregate meal programs, transportation services, counseling services (alcohol abuse, depression, bereavement, etc.), home health care agencies, day care programs, etc.

Please repeat this screen at least once each year--sooner if the individual has a major change in his or her health, income, immediate family (e.g., spouse dies), or functional status.

These materials developed by the Nutrition Screening Initiative

*Make relevant adjustment by country.

Using the Level I Screen

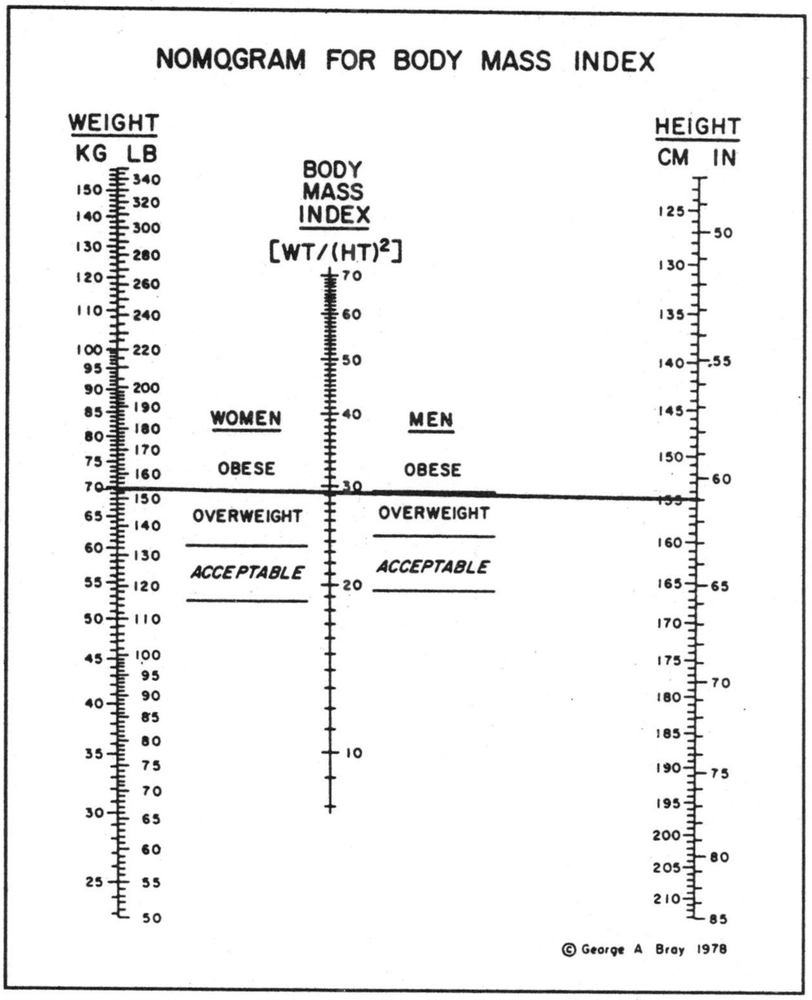

Body Weight

Because our bodies reflect how much and what we eat, measuring height and weight is one of the simplest but most important ways of monitoring nutritional status. This information can then be used to assess quickly whether the individual is over- or underweight with the Body Mass Index (BMI) scale.

The National Research Council's Committee on Diet and Health has suggested that persons over 65 should have a BMI of 24 to 29. Values below 24 indicate that the individual may be ill, malnourished, or both and should therefore seek medical attention. Values above 29 indicate that the individual is obese and is at risk for (or may already have) high blood pressure, diabetes, or osteoarthritis. The upper limit for screening older adults is 27, which represents high risk for obesity; the risk for becoming obese starts at 25.

In the example to the right, the individual is 5'1" tall (61") and weighs 153 lbs. The BMI is just about 29, which indicates that the individual should be referred to a physician for medical treatment.

Keeping track of height and weight over time is also helpful, since rapid weight loss usually means the person is already sick or is trying to fight off a disease. Rapid weight gain may also be caused by illness and often brings on a number of health disorders. Even when weight change is associated with an emotional cause (such as depression due to the death of a spouse), the health consequences are significant. If the individual has lost or gained weight in the past few months, he or she should see a health care professional for a check-up.

Eating Habits

Obviously, what the individual eats from day to day will greatly affect his or her nutritional status and overall health. An older adult may appear to be the right weight and to look well, but if he or she regularly omits an entire category of food, the risk for specific diseases increases tremendously. Even overweight individuals may (and often do) eat a diet that does not supply the body with enough nutrients. For example, only 13% of adults aged 55 to 74 years eat enough fruits and vegetables! It is especially important that older Americans consume milk products, fruits, and vegetables on a daily basis since these foods supply them with vitamins and minerals that are critical to maintaining their health.

Following are the U.S. Dietary Guidelines, which were just revised in 1990. You may want to ask friends, family members, or other persons who interact with this individual whether he or she eats foods from each of the food groups on a daily basis and how frequently he or she has meals and snacks. If the individual is on a special diet prescribed by a health care professional, stress the importance of following the instructions closely. Older adults who restrict their diet may benefit from nutrition education to clear up any misconceptions they might have about specific foods.

Persons who have trouble eating a healthy diet should be referred to a registered dietitian, who can offer individual nutrition education and assist them with selecting nutritious foods that they can enjoy, afford, prepare, and digest easily. For those who have difficulty eating food, the dietitian may recommend nutrition intervention that could include medical nutritionals. Those who often find that they do not have sufficient food or who go entire days without eating should be referred to a social service worker to identify local resources (food stamps, meal programs, other assistance).

Persons who drink alcohol almost every day are at risk for nutritional and health problems and should seek professional treatment for alcohol abuse.

Persons who consistently neglect to meet the minimum number of servings (right) for several months should see their physician to determine whether they have developed any serious health problems as a result of their poor diet.

U.S. Dietary Guidelines (Revised 1990)

Eat a variety of foods.
3-5 servings vegetables (especially dark green & yellow)
2-4 servings fruits (especially citrus)
6-11 servings breads, cereals, rice, pasta
2-3 servings milk, yogurt, cheese
2-3 servings meats, poultry, fish, dry beans & peas, eggs, nuts

Maintain healthy weight.
Choose a diet low in fat, saturated fat, and cholesterol.
<30% of daily calories from fat
<10% of daily calories from saturated fat
<300 mg cholesterol per day

Choose a diet with plenty of vegetables, fruits, and grain products.
1 serving veg/fruit = 1 c raw, 1/2 c cooked, 1 med piece
1 serving grain = 1 sl bread, 1/2 bun, bagel, Engl. muffin, 1 oz cold cereal, 1/2 c cooked cereal, rice, pasta, grains

Use sugars in moderation only.
Examples of sugars include: table sugar, brown sugar, raw sugar, glucose, fructose, maltose, lactose, honey, syrup, corn sweetener, high-fructose corn syrup, molasses, fruit juice concentrate

Use salt and sodium in moderation only.
1,100-3,300 mg sodium daily

If you drink alcoholic beverages, do so in moderation.
<1 drink/day for women, <2 drinks/day for men
1 drink = 12 oz beer, 5 oz wine, 1.5 oz liquor (80 proof)

U.S. Department of Agriculture, U.S. Department of Health and Human Services. Nutrition and Your Health: Dietary Guidelines for Americans. Third Edition. Home and Garden Bulletin No. 232. Washington, DC: U.S. Government Printing Office, 1990.

Living Environment

Screening for income and social activity, while not specific indicators of poor nutritional status, can identify significant risk factors for malnutrition. Approximately 17% of men and 42% of women aged 65 and older reported incomes of less than $6,000 in 1990; individuals who spend less than $30 per week on food probably do not meet the recommended dietary allowances for many nutrients. Individuals who have an unreliable source of income, who have recently experienced a loss of income, or who rely on economic assistance programs are at risk for poor nutritional status and should therefore be monitored carefully, with extra attention paid to changes in body weight and eating habits.

Older persons who live alone may also find it difficult to shop for or cook food or may simply lack the motivation to prepare food - especially if they have recently lost a family member, a friend, or their own independence (due to loss of ability to walk, drive, take a taxi or public transportation, or perform other routine activities). A person in this situation probably can't buy or prepare enough food and may therefore develop health problems as a result of poor nutritional status. And even if they are functioning well, many older Americans do not have working refrigerators or stoves for food storage and preparation, which severely limits their diet.

Functional Status

Decline in functional status represents one of the most important "symptoms" of nutritional and overall health to be monitored in any older population. Two measures of dependence are commonly used to assess functional status: Activities of Daily Living (ADLs), which measure very basic self-care activities, and Instrumental Activities of Daily Living (IADLs), which measure home-management activities that are essential to independent living. Not surprisingly, difficulties with personal care activities (ADLs) increase with age, though the ability to eat is affected to a lesser extent than is walking or bathing. Problems in conducting more complex daily activities (IADLs), including social functioning and home management activities, affect a larger percentage of older Americans, particularly among adults over age 85.

The inability to perform any of the six activities of daily living (ADLs) and the nutrition-related instrumental activities of daily living (IADLs) signals a high level of dependence and the potential presence of disease as well as of poor nutritional status. The tables below list the ADLs and the IADLs and describe the difference between independence and dependence for all ADLs and the three nutrition-related IADLs (which relate more closely to nutritional status than the others).

Activities of Daily Living (ADLs)

Bathing. Independent: assistance only in bathing a single part (back or disabled extremity) or bathes self completely. Dependent: assistance in bathing more than one part of body; assistance getting in or out of tub; does not bathe self

Dressing. Independent: gets clothes from closets & drawers; puts on clothes, outer garments, braces; manages fasteners (act of tying shoes is excluded). Dependent: does not dress self or remains partly undressed

Toileting. Independent: gets to toilet; gets on & off toilet; arranges clothes; cleans organs of excretion; may manage own bedpan used at night only: may or may not use mechanical supports. Dependent: uses bedpan or commode or receives assistance getting to & using toilet

Transferring. Independent: moves in & out of bed independently; moves in & out of chair independently; may or may not use mechanical support. Dependent: assistance in moving in or out of bed and/or chair; does not perform one or more transfers

Continence. Independent: urination & defecation entirely self-controlled. Dependent: partial or total incontinence in urination or defecation; partial or total control by enemas, catheters, or regulated use of urinals and/or bedpans

Feeding. Independent: gets food from plate or its equivalent into mouth (precutting of meat & preparation of food, such as buttering bread, are excluded). Dependent: assistance in act of feeding; does not eat at all or parenteral feeding.

Modified from Katz S, Downs TD, Cash HR, Grotz RC. Progress in the development of the index of the ADL. Gerontologist 1970; 10:20-30. © 1969 The Gerontological Society of America. Reprinted with permission.

Instrumental Activities of Daily Living (IADLs)

Ability to Use Telephone

Shopping.* Independent: takes care of all shopping needs; shops independently for small purchases. Dependent: must be accompanied on any shopping trip; completely unable to shop.

Food Preparation.* Independent: plans, prepares, & serves adequate meals independently; prepares adequate meals if supplied with ingredients. Dependent: heats & serves prepared meals; prepares meals but does not maintain adequate diet; must have meals prepared & served

Housekeeping

Laundry

Mode of Transportation.* Independent: travels independently on public transportation or drives own car; arranges own travel via taxi but does not otherwise use public transportation. Dependent: travels on public transportation when assisted or accompanied by another; travel limited to taxi or automobile with assistance; does not travel at all.

Responsibility for Own Medication

Ability to Handle Finances

**Nutrition-related IADL. Modified from Lawton MP, Brody EM. Assessment of older people: self-monitoring and instrumental activities of daily living. Gerontologist 1969; 179-186. © 1970 The Gerontological Society of America. Reprinted with permission.*

Summary

Most older adults with whom you interact will have a few existing or potential risk factors for poor nutritional status, but they will also probably be able to address these issues themselves with minimal (but appropriate) assistance. Many would benefit from an appointment with a registered dietitian, which may be a new concept to them. Others may need to see health care and social service professionals with whom they are accustomed to visiting, such as their dentist, their case worker, or a counseling service. Finally, some will need to see a physician for a complete examination. Many people don't think of poor diet or changes in body weight as a sufficient cause for seeking medical attention, but we hope to alert all Americans, particularly those who are older, to the critical role played by nutrition in maintaining good health and in preventing disease.

Overview

Everyone wants some of your time, and already there's barely enough time allotted to the typical medical examination to perform even a routine checkup. How can you possibly fit one more screen in?

We hope it will be easy. Most of the information on this screen is already obtained during a routine physical or is available in the patient chart. Some questions can be asked while the patient is waiting in the reception area or in an examination room. Other statements will have been previously flagged on the Nutritional Health Checklist or the Level I Screen (or both). Chances are that you will only need to add a few additional questions to your usual patient interview to complete a Level II Screen, which can be done in coordination with other staff members. At the very least, pay close attention to changes in body weight and height and, when blood work is done, to serum albumin.

Of course, not everyone needs a Level II Screen. Patients could be given the Nutritional Health Checklist in the waiting room before you see them; if they have any questions or concerns, you'll probably be able to prevent today a bigger nutritional or medical problem that would otherwise bring them back to your office in a few months. If they've marked a risk factor that merits further attention, such as alcohol abuse or chronically inadequate nutritional intake, you could make an appropriate referral.

Please familiarize yourself with the content of both the Level I and Level II Screens. Some information is duplicated on the two screens so that you have the option of skipping the Level I Screen without missing any important risk factors. If you already use patient assessment forms and would rather not add more paperwork to the chart, please consider adding a brief section on nutrition screening based on these tools. Finally, if you are unfamiliar with some of the measurements used (e.g., circumferences, skinfolds, mini-mental examination, depression screening, etc.), their use is explained briefly in this manual. The Nutrition Screening Initiative offers workshops and additional information on performing these assessments; please contact the Initiative for information on the dates and locations of such workshops.

Level II Screen

Complete the following screen by interviewing the patient directly and/or by referring to the patient chart. If you do not routinely perform all of the described tests or ask all of the listed questions, please consider including them but do not be concerned if the entire screen is not completed. Please try to collect serial measurements, which are extremely valuable in monitoring nutritional status. Please refer to the manual for additional information.

Anthropometrics

Measure height to the nearest inch and weight to the nearest or pound or kg. Record the values below and mark them on the Body Mass Index (BMI) scale to the right. Then use a straight edge (paper, ruler) connect the two points and circle the spot where this straight line crosses the center line (body mass index). Record the number below; healthy older adults should have a BMI between 24 and 27; check the appropriate box to flag an abnormally high or low value.

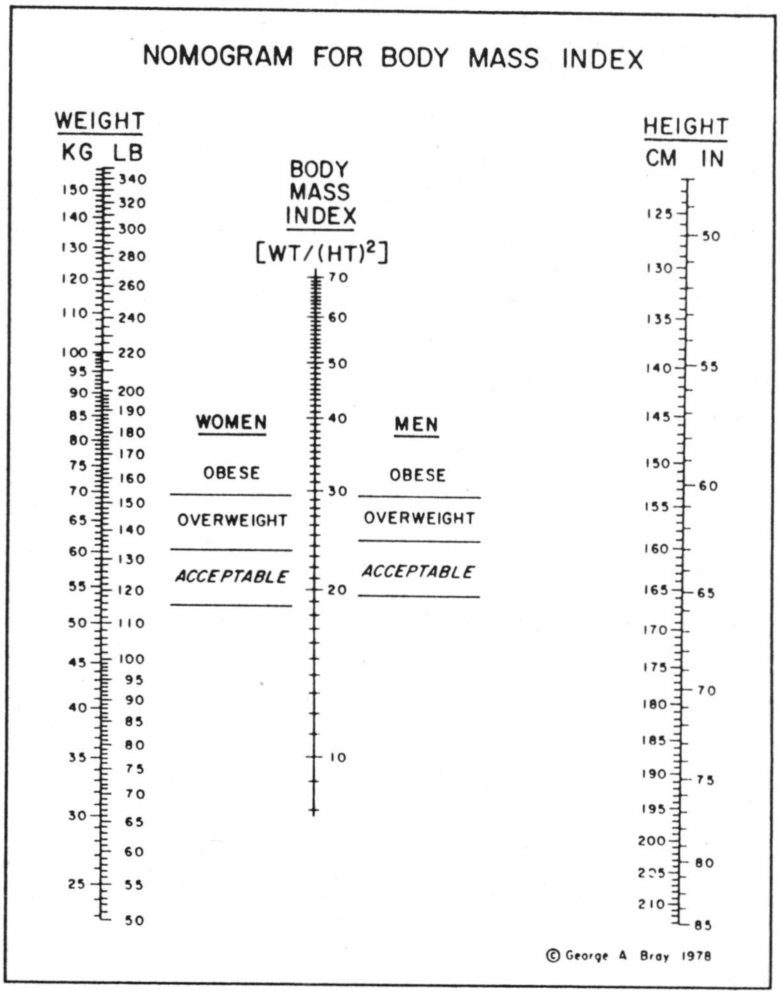

Height (in/cm):______________
Weight (lbs/kg):_____________
Body Mass Index
(weight/height):_____________

Please place a check by any statement regarding BMI and recent weight loss that is true for the patient.

- ❑ Body mass index <24
- ❑ Body mass index >27
- ❑ Has lost or gained 10 pounds or 4.5 kg (or more) of body weight in the past 6 months

Record the measurement of mid-arm circumference to the nearest 0.1 centimeter and of triceps skinfold to the nearest 2 millimeters.

Mid-Arm Circumference (cm):___________
Triceps Skinfold (mm):________________
Mid-Arm Muscle Circumference (cm):_____

Refer to the table and check any abnormal values:

- ❑ Mid-arm muscle circumference <10th percentile
- ❑ Triceps skinfold <10th percentile
- ❑ Triceps skinfold >95th percentile

Note mid-arm circumference (cm) - 0.314 x triceps skinfold (mm) = mid-arm *muscle* circumference (cm)

For the remaining sections, please place a check by any statements that are true for the patient.

Laboratory Data

(normal values used by national hospital will need to be used)

- ❑ Serum albumin below 3.5 g/dl
- ❑ Serum cholesterol below 160 mg/dl
- ❑ Serum cholesterol above 240 mg/dl

Drug Use

- ❑ Three or more prescription drugs, OTC medications, and/or vitamin/mineral supplements daily

Clinical Features

Presence of (check each that apply):

- ❑ Problems with mouth, teeth, or gums
- ❑ Difficulty chewing
- ❑ Difficulty swallowing
- ❑ Angular stomatitis
- ❑ Glossitis
- ❑ History of bone pain
- ❑ History of bone fractures
- ❑ Skin canges (dry, loose, nonspecific lesions, edema)

Percentile	Men 55-65 y	Men 65-75 y	Women 55-65 y	Women 65-75 y
Arm circumference (cm)				
10th	27.3	26.3	25.7	25.2
50th	31.7	30.7	30.3	29.9
95th	36.9	35.5	38.5	37.3
Arm muscle circumference (cm)				
10th	24.5	23.5	19.6	19.5
50th	27.8	26.8	22.5	22.5
95th	32.0	30.6	28.0	27.9
Triceps skinfold (mm)				
10th	6	6	16	14
50th	11	11	25	24
95th	22	22	38	36

From: Frisancho AR. New norms of upper limb fat and muscle areas for assessment of nutritional status. Am J Clin Nutr 1981; 34:2540-2545. © *1981 American Society for Clinical Nutrition.*

Eating Habits

- ❑ Does not have enough food to eat each day
- ❑ Usually eats alone
- ❑ Does not eat anything on one or more days each month
- ❑ Has poor appetite
- ❑ Is on a special diet
- ❑ Eats vegetables two or fewer times daily
- ❑ Eats milk or milk products once or not at all daily
- ❑ Eats fruit or drinks fruit juice once or not at all daily
- ❑ Eats breads, cereals, pasta, rice, or other grains five or fewer times daily
- ❑ Has more than one alcoholic drink per day (if woman); more than two drinks per day (if man)

Living Environment

- ❑ Lives on an income of less than $6000 per year (per individual in the household or appropriate figure for your country)
- ❑ Lives alone
- ❑ Is housebound
- ❑ Is concerned about home security
- ❑ Lives in a home with inadeaquate heating or cooling
- ❑ Does not have a stove and/or refrigerator
- ❑ Is unable or prefers not to spend enough money on food

Functional Status

Usually or always needs assistance with (check each that apply):

- ❑ Bathing
- ❑ Dressing
- ❑ Grooming
- ❑ Toileting
- ❑ Eating
- ❑ Walking or moving about
- ❑ Traveling (outside the home)
- ❑ Preparing food
- ❑ Shopping for food or other necessities

Mental/Cognitive Status

- ❑ Clinical evidence of impairment, e.g. Folstein<26
- ❑ Clinical evidence of depressive illness, e.g. Beck Depression Inventory>15, Geriatric Depression Scale>5

Patients in whom you have identified or more major indicator (see page 2) of poor nutritional status require immediate medical attention; if minor indicators are found, ensure that they are known to a health professional or to the patient's own physician. Patients who display risk factors (see page 2) of poor nutritional status should be referred to the appropriate health care or social service professional (dietitian, nurse, dentist, case manager, etc.).

These materials developed by the Nutrition Screening Initiative.

Using the Level II Screen

Men: 64.19 (0.04 x age) + (2.02 x knee height)
Women: 84.88 - (0.24 x age) + (1.83 x knee height)

Height Estimate: measure knee height (inches) from the bottom of the foot to the anterior of the knee with the ankle and the knee at 90^0; measure age in years. These standards probably do not apply to non-Caucasians.

Chumlea WC, Roch AF, Mukherjee D. Nutritional assessment of the elderly through anthropometry. Columbus, OH: Ross Laboratories, 1984.

Anthropometrics (see also p 9, Level I Screen)

Changes in body weight and composition reflect dietary intake and serve as general indicators of nutritional and overall health. Please review information presented on page 7 as well as the following points.

Kyphosis and scoliosis may make the measurement of height difficult in older adults, but an estimate is essential to determine body mass index and to monitor bone loss. The equations to the right can be used to estimate the height of bedridden patients as well as those who are unable to stand erect.

Loss of height is an early indicator of osteoporosis, which is a major nutritional disease among older adults. If the recorded height is 2 to 3 inches less than the patient had estimated, or if serial height measurements indicate a loss, steps should be taken to intervene and prevent further bone loss.

Body mass index (BMI) is a weight-to-height ratio that is also highly correlated with body fat; BMI is calculated by dividing body weight (kg) by height-squared (m^2). Individuals who have a BMI below 24 or who are 80% or less of their desirable body weight for height are at increased risk for disease and for poor nutritional status. At the other extreme, persons who have a BMI above 27 or who are 120% or more of their desirable body weight have developed obesity, which is a medically significant disease, and are at very increased risk for a number of related conditions (hypertension, diabetes, osteoarthritis). Older adults with a BMI of 25 or 26 are also at risk for developing obesity and its comorbidity and should receive appropriate intervention as well.

Large or sudden change in body weight, whether gained or lost, could indicate the imminence or presence of disease, and the medical cause should be investigated promptly (particularly severe weight loss). Even when weight change is associated with an emotional cause (e.g., depression), the health consequences are significant.

Because this is a screening tool, the use of two anthropometric variables to define either obesity or undernutrition is not essential, and, due to the potential for errors in measurement, values should be treated as estimates. However, by measuring mid-arm circumferences and/or tricep skinfolds, the risk of misclassification is reduced significantly. Skinfold values can be used to assess subcutaneous fat levels, which may in turn indicate the presence of obesity or protein-calorie malnutrition. Mid-arm circumference can be used to indicate both calorie and protein stores, although depressed values are usually found only in persons with severe malnutrition. Mid-arm muscle circumference may serve as a more sensitive indicator of body protein reserves. The Initiative would hope that you would use this opportunity to become familiar with these important skills for assessing nutritional status quickly and efficiently.

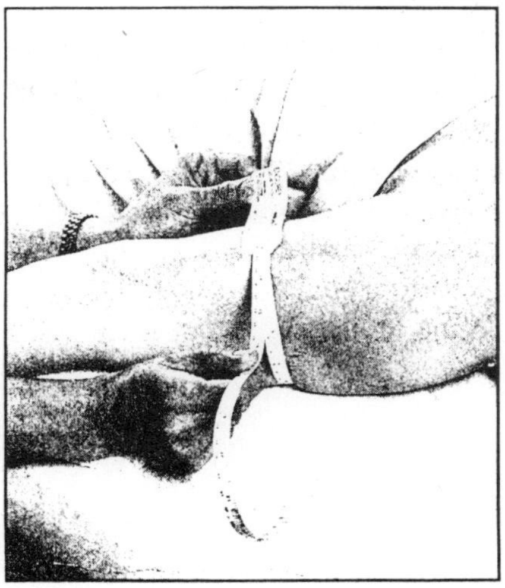

To measure mid-arm circumference (left), place a flexible tape midway between the tip of the acromial process of the scapula and the olecranon process of the ulna; hold the tape firmly but gently to avoid compressing the soft tissue.

To measure triceps skinfold (right), grasp double fold of skin at the same midpoint used to measure circumference and place the caliper jaws perpendicular to the length of skinfold.

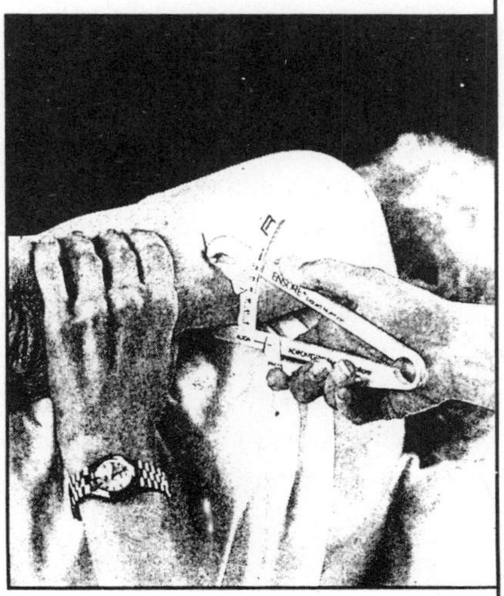

Laboratory Data

Albumin, with its 17- to 20-day half-life, is sensitive to changes in nutritional status. Although many factors can modify serum levels, albumin remains an economic and potentially useful indicator of poor nutritional status and protein malnutrition. Similarly, total cholesterol can indicate poor nutrition at both extremes: levels below 160 mg/dl have been associated with increased mortality in nursing home populations, and levels above 240 mg/dl have been identified as high risk by the National Cholesterol Education Program. Many other parameters of routine blood and urine testing can be also used to screen older Americans for nutritional disorders, such as folate, iron, ascorbic acid, and zinc; laboratory values less specific to nutritional disorders include complete blood count, total lymphocyte count, thyroid tests, electrolytes, vitamins A and B12, and BUN/creatinine.

Drug Use

Chronic use of over-the-counter or prescribed medication can significantly affect nutritional status. Not only is the potential for adverse drug-nutrient interactions high, but poor nutritional status can alter drug absorption, metabolism, or utilization. Because polypharmacy is so prevalent among older adults, patients must be interviewed carefully to ensure full and accurate reporting of all prescription and over-the-counter medications. In addition, many older Americans use vitamin/mineral supplements, which are not a substitute for a healthy and balanced diet, and which may be toxic when consumed in amounts that dramatically and/or chronically exceed the recommended dietary allowances. While no major indicators of poor nutritional status are directly related to medication use, the concurrent use of multiple medications represents an indicator of poor nutritional status, and the risk for a number of potential adverse interactions must be monitored.

Clinical Features

A nutrition-related physical examination may confirm significant weight change or unhealthy body weight (whether over- or underweight). Many signs found on physical examination are likely to be associated with, and thus to indicate, poor nutritional status. A thorough oral examination may identify signs of vitamin B and C deficiencies (cheilosis, glossitis, angular stomatitis), dehydration, and risk factors for poor nutritional status, such as ill-fitting dentures, bleeding gums, caries, loose teeth, and xerostomia. Dysphagia also represents an important minor indicator of poor nutritional status; in addition to having patients swallow to assess mobility of the thyroid gland, evaluate their ability to swallow both fluids and solids.

Bone tenderness and back pain are associated with osteoporosis and in turn with potential calcium, vitamin D, and sunlight deficiencies. When examining for bone loss, note also the presence of muscular strength and mass; muscular wasting may indicate poor nutritional status, and reduced strength and range of motion can impair functional ability, particularly with regard to food preparation.

Evidence of subcutaneous fat loss and dryness of the skin should be sought as well. Floppy, loose skin and striae indicate weight loss. Nonspecific lesions are indicators of poor nutritional status. Fluid retention may indicate protein deficiency or renal, cardiac or hepatic disease.

Eating Habits (see also pp 9-10, Level I Screen)

Unfortunately, assessing dietary intake in older adults can be difficult due to impaired recall and reduced appetite. More reliable information may be obtained from individuals who interact with the patient on a social or caregiving basis. Compare information from all available sources on the specific number of food servings consumed with dietary recommendations (listed on page 10), particularly with regard to intake of fruits, vegetables, and dairy products. If one or more food groups has been chronically omitted from the patient's diet, pay close attention to clinical features related to specific deficiencies. Assessment by a registered dietitian is important for nutritional care planning when nutrition problems are present. Referral to a registered dietitian can be done if no one is available in the setting.

In addition to the guidelines presented on pages 9 and 10, review the patient's chart for other symptoms that may indicate poor nutritional status: anorexia, early satiety, nausea, vomiting, dyspepsia, constipation, diarrhea, and dehydration. Interview the patient about any sensory impairment that might be directly (reduced ability to taste or smell) or indirectly (loss of visual acuity) affecting his/her dietary intake as well.

Living Environment (see also p 10, Level I Screen)

Significant changes in psychosocial status are risk factors for poor nutritional status, which in turn can induce psychosocial changes. Review the issues regarding income and social isolation discussed on page 10. Ask the patient about recent bereavement, recent relocation or discharge from a hospital or rehabilitation center, financial difficulties, neighborhood crime, or any other factors that, by interrupting the older patient's habits, may upset the nutritional schedule and routine.

Functional Status (see also p 10-11, Level I Screen)

The role of functional status in geriatric medicine cannot be overstated. Any decline in self-care (ADLs) or home-management (IADLs) activities should be regarded as both a risk factor for and an indicator of poor nutritional status. Both the Activities of Daily Living (bathing, dressing, toileting, transferring, continence, feeding) and the Instrumental Activities of Daily Living (use telephone, shopping, food preparation, housekeeping, laundry, mode of transportation, manage own medications, manage finances) are reviewed on page 11; guidelines for distinguishing between independence and dependence for specific tasks are also provided. When interviewing patients, family members, friends, and other caregivers, define "dependence" as "needing assistance for that activity most of the time" and "independence" as "can be performed without assistance". Pay particular attention to changes in the functional status of IADLs that relate to the likelihood of the patient obtaining, preparing, and eating an adequate diet (i.e., shopping, food preparation, and mode of transportation).

Mini-Mental State Examination

Orientation: Ask for the date (What is the year / season / date / day / month?). Ask specifically for parts omitted (e.g., Can you also tell me what season it is?). Give 1 point for each correct (0-5).
Ask in turn, Can you tell me the name of this hospital? (floor, town, county, state). Give 1 point for each correct (0-5).

Registration: Ask the patient if you may test his memory. Then say the names of 3 unrelated objects, (i.e. ball, tree, flag) clearly and slowly, about one second for each. After you have said all three, ask him or her to repeat them. This first repetition determines his score (0-3), but keep saying them until he can repeat all three, up to six trials. If he does not eventually learn all three, recall cannot be meaningfully tested.

Attention & Calculation: Ask the patient to begin with 100 and count backward by 7. Stop after 5 subtractions (93, 86, 79, 72, 65). Score the total number of correct answers (0-5).
If the patient cannot or will not perform this task, ask him to spell the word "world" backward. The score is the number of letters in correct order (e.g., dlrow = 5; dlorw = 3).

Recall: Ask the patient if he can recall the 3 objects you previously asked him to remember. Score 0-3.

Language:

Naming: Show the patient a wrist watch and ask him what it is. Repeat for a pencil. Score 0-2.
Repetition: Ask the patient to repeat the following sentence: "No ifs, ands, or buts". Allow only one trial. Score 0 or 1.
3-Stage Command: Ask the patient to follow a 3-stage command: "Take a paper in your right hand, fold it in half, and put it on the floor". Score 1 point for each part correctly executed (0-3).
Reading: On a blank piece of paper, print the sentence "Close your eyes" in letters large enough for the patient to see clearly. Ask him to read it and do what it says. Score 1 point only if he actually closes his eyes.
Writing: Give the patient a blank piece of paper and ask him to write a sentence for you. Do not dictate a sentence. It is to be written spontaneously. It must contain a subject and a verb and be sensible, though correct grammar and punctuation are not necessary (0-1).
Copying: On a clean piece of paper, draw intersecting pentagons (1" sides) and ask the patient to copy it exactly as it is. All 10 angles must be present, and 2 must intersect to score 1 point. Tremor and rotation are ignored.

Assess level of consciousness along a continuum:

Alert — Drowsy — Stupor — Coma

From: Folstein MF, Folstein SE, McHugh PR. Mini-Mental State: a practical guide for grading the cognitive state of patients for the clinician. J Psychiat Res 1975; 12:189-198.

Geriatric Depression Scale

Choose the best answer for how you felt over the past week.

1. Are you basically satisfied with your life? yes/no
2. Have you dropped many of your activities and interests? yes/no
3. Do you feel that your life is empty? yes/no
4. Do you often get bored? yes/no
5. Are you hopeful about the future? yes/no
6. Are you bothered by thoughts that you can't get out of your head? yes/no
7. Are you in good spirits most of the time? yes/no
8. Are you afraid that something bad is going to happen to you? yes/no
9. Do you feel happy most of the time? yes/no
10. Do you often feel helpless? yes/no
11. Do you often get restless and fidgety? yes/no
12. Do you prefer to stay at home, rather than going out doing new things? yes/no
13. Do you frequently worry about the future? yes/no
14. Do you feel you have more problems with your memory than most? yes/no
15. Do you think it is wonderful to be alive now? yes/no
16. Do you often feel downhearted and blue? yes/no
17. Do you feel pretty worthless the way you are now? yes/no
18. Do you worry a lot about the past? yes/no
19. Do you find life very exciting? yes/no
20. Is it hard for you to get started on new projects? yes/no
21. Do you feel full of energy? yes/no
22. Do you feel that your situation is hopeless? yes/no
23. Do you think that most people are better off than you are? yes/no
24. Do you frequently get upset over little things? yes/no
25. Do you frequently feel like crying? yes/no
26. Do you have trouble concentrating? yes/no
27. Do you enjoy getting up in the morning? yes/no
28. Do you prefer to avoid social gatherings? yes/no
29. Is it easy for you to make decisions? yes/no
30. Is your mind as clear as it used to be? yes/no

From: Yesavage JA, Brink TL, Rose TL, Lum O, Huang V, Adey M, Leirer VO. Development and validation of a geriatric depression screening scale: a preliminary report. J Psychiat Res 1983; 17:37-49.

Mental/Cognitive Status (see also pp 17-18, 20)

Just as change in functional status can indicate a number of disease processes as well as poor nutritional status, diminished or changed cognitive status can serve as both an indicator of and risk factor for nutritional disorders. Cognitive status refers to the patient's intellectual capability, including such testable areas as memory, language, math, abstraction, reading, writing, and orientation to time, place, and person. Dementia, which is responsible for most loss of cognitive function, has been associated with B12 deficiency, and dementias and depression caused by metabolic disorders, drug toxicity, hypothyroidism, and confusion are likely to be associated with malnutrition. Some mental illness can also result from dehydration and protein energy malnutrition.

Physicians involved in geriatric medicine have long been encouraged to employ mental status instruments in clinical practice. While the use of such instruments does require some training, one of the most widely validated short instruments (Folstein Mini-Mental State Examination, p 17) has been validated using trained high school students. The mean score in the validation studies for normal subjects on this instrument was 27.6. Clinical experience has shown that a score of less than 26 is abnormal, and could lead to, or have resulted from, poor nutritional state. A score of less than 26 should anyway be regarded as indicating a strong possibility of dementia, and the attention of a physician should be sought to ensure that the many other illnesses that can result in cognitive decline have been considered. This would include depression, which in older individuals will frequently reduce the score on such a test. As with anthropometric measurements, cognitive status is best monitored serially.

Depression itself, whether the term is used loosely to mean a state of sadness or loss of interest or used in a clinical sense, should be regarded as an indicator of poor nutritional status. Screening for major depression and melancholia will identify patients who would benefit from specific medical treatment to reduce self-neglect as well as the risk of suicide. This manual includes two short screens on pages 18 and 20: the Geriatric Depression Scale (GDS) and the Beck Depression Inventory (BDI). On the 30-question (yes/no) GDS, 20 questions indicate the presence of depression when answered positively, while the remaining 10 (#1, 5, 7, 9, 15,19, 21, 27, 29, and 30) indicate depression when answered negatively. The GDS has been shown to be a reliable and valid measure of geriatric depression with a high degree of internal consistency. Sensitivity and specificity studies have suggested that scores of 0-10 be considered normal, while 11 or greater indicate possible depression.

The BDI (short form) is a 13-item questionnaire that the patient can complete in about five minutes. Scores of 0-4 indicate no or minimal depression; of 5-7 indicate mild depression; of 8-15 indicate moderate depression; and of 16 or greater indicate severe depression. This scale was devised to screen family practice patients and is not specific to older adults (as the GDS is) and may be difficult for a cognitively impaired older person to complete, but its validity and reliability are well documented.

Instruments for assessing mental and cognitive status as well as depression are provided on the following pages.

Summary

Please remember to treat the Level II Screen as a screening rather than a diagnostic device. Information obtained on the screen may be used to develop a final diagnosis, but the more essential goal is to start looking for signs of nutritional deficiencies and disorders. By initiating an efficient and systematic method of screening for poor nutritional status, you will have taken an important step in improving the health and well-being of your patients without adding a significant drain on your resources. In fact, you will almost certainly save your and -your patients' time and money down the road.

Beck Depression Inventory-Short Form

This is a questionnaire. On the questionnaire are groups of statements. Please read the entire group of statements in each category. Then pick out the one statement in that group which best describes the way you feel today, that is, right now! Circle the number beside the statement you have chosen. If several statements in the group seem to apply equally well, circle each one.

Be sure to read all the statements in each group before making your choice.

A.(Sadness)
3 I am so sad or unhappy that I can't stand it.
2 I am so blue or sad all the time and I can't snap out of it.
1 I feel sad or blue.
0 I do not feel sad.

B.(Pessimism)
3 I feel that the future is hopeless and that things cannot improve.
2 I feel I have nothing to look forward to.
1 I feel discouraged about the future.
0 I am not particularly pessimistic or discouraged about the future.

C.(Sense of Failure)
3 I feel I am a complete failure as a person (parent, husband, wife).
2 As I look back on my life, all I can see is a lot of failures.
1 I feel I have failed more than the average person.
0 I do not feel like a failure.

D.(Dissatisfaction)
3 I am dissatisfied with everything.
2 I don't get satisfaction out of anything anymore.
1 I don't enjoy things the way I used to.
0 I am not particularly dissatisfied.

E. (Guilt)
3 I feel as though I am very bad or worthless.
2 I feel quite guilty.
1 I feel bad or unworthy a good part of the time.
0 I don't feel particularly guilty.

F. (Self-Dislike)
3 I hate myself.
2 I am disgusted with myself.
1 I am disappointed with myself.
0 I don't feel disappointed in myself.

G.(Self-Harm)
3 I would kill myself if I had the chance.
2 I have definite plans about committing suicide.
1 I feel I would be better off dead.
0 I don't have any thoughts of harming myself.

H.(Social Withdrawal)
3 I have lost all of my interest in other people and don't care about them at all.
2 I have lost most of my interest in other people and have little feeling for them.
1 I am less interested in other people than I used to be.
0 I have not lost interest in other people.

I. (Indecisiveness)
3 I can't make any decisions at all anymore.
2 I have great difficulty in making decisions.
1 I try to put off making decisions.
0 I make decisions as well as ever.

J. (Self-Image Change)
3 I feel that I am ugly or repulsive looking.
2 I feel that there are permanent changes in my appearance and they make me look unattractive.
1 I am worried that I am looking old or unattractive.
0 I don't feel that I look any worse than I used to.

K.(Work Difficulty)
3 I can't do any work at all.
2 I have to push myself very hard to do anything.
1 It takes an extra effort to get started at doing something.
0 I can work about as well as before.

L.(Fatigability)
3 I get too tired to do anything.
2 I get tired from doing anything.
1 I get tired more easily than I used to.
0 I don't get any more tired than usual.

M.(Anorexia)
3 I have no appetite at all anymore.
2 My appetite is much worse now.
1 My appetite is not as good as it used to be.
0 My appetite is no worse than usual.

From: Beck AT, Beck RW. Screening depressed patients in family practice: a rapid technic. Postgrad Med 1972; Dec:81-85.

Summary of Nutrition Screening

"DETERMINE Your Nutritional Health" Checklist (self-administered)
- Public awareness tool/nutritional health checklist

Level I Screen (administered in any setting)
- Administered by community member, social worker, or health care professional
- Administered to individuals with identified warning signs (from Nutritional Health Checklist)

Level II Screen (administered in health care setting)
- Administered by physician or other qualified health care professional
- Followup to abnormal Level I Screen and/or Nutritional Health Checklist

Self-Help
- No major indicators of poor nutritional status, no or few minor indicators or risk factors
- Clear understanding of and willingness to improve diet/lifestyle

Referral to Other Social Service and Health Care Professionals as Appropriate
- Case Worker
- Counselor
- Dentist
- Dietitian
- Home Health Care Agent
- Meal Program Administrator
- Nurse
- Pharmacist
- Psychologist
- Social Worker

Medical Intervention
- >10% weight loss in last 6 months (5% loss in 1 month, 7.5% in 3 months)
- BMI <24 or >27 (<80% or >120% of desirable body weight)
- Triceps skinfold below 10th percentile or above 95th percentile
- Mid-arm muscle circumference below 10th percentile
- Serum albumin <3.5 g/dl
- Change from independent to dependent in 2 ADLs or in 1 nutrition-related IADL
- >3 months of failure to consume diet that meets the U.S. Dietary Guidelines
- Presence of osteoporosis, osteomalacia, folate deficiency, or B12 deficiency

SCHEMATIC- A PRACTICAL APPPROACH TO NUTRITIONAL SCREENING

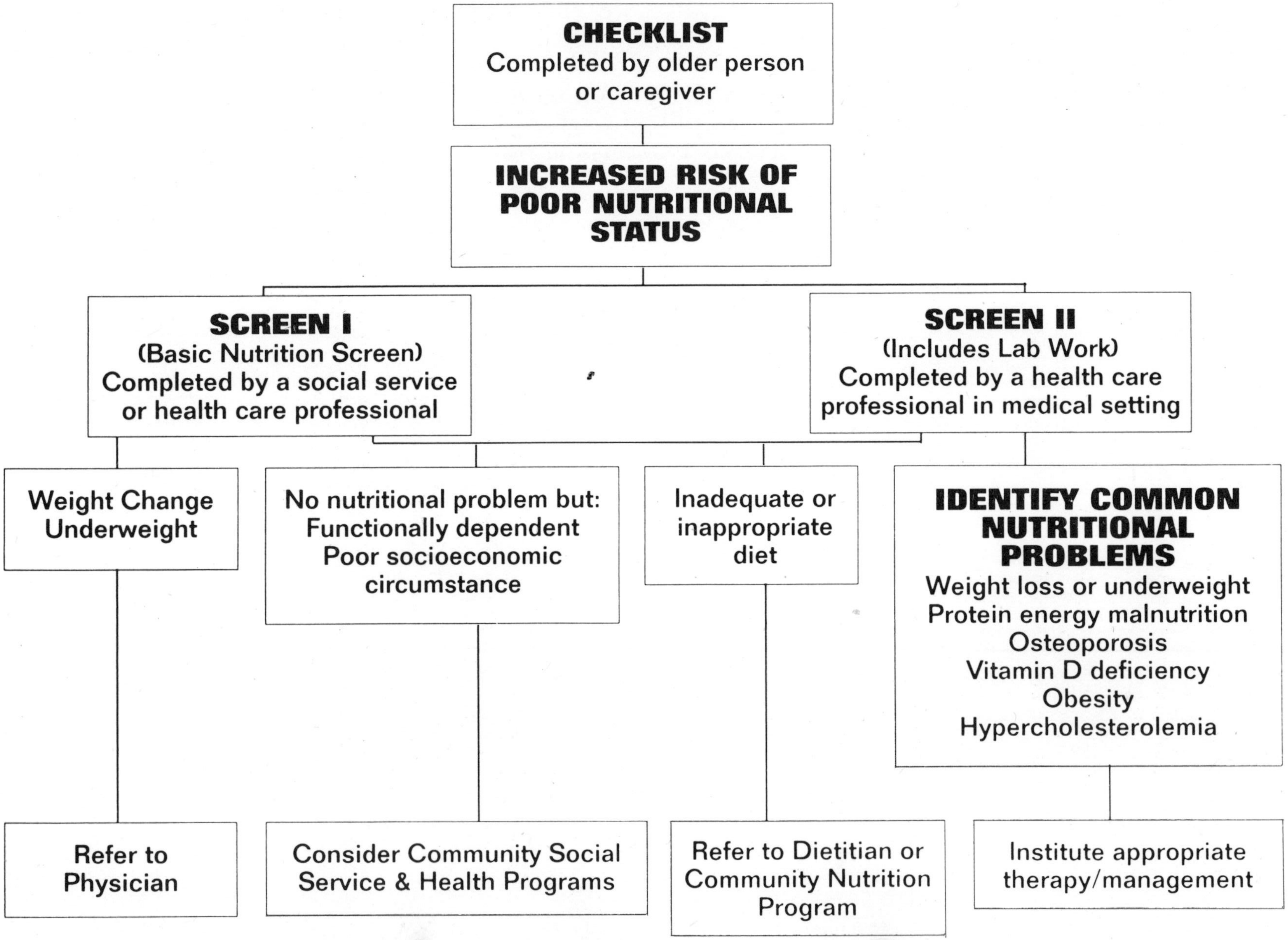

Options for Intervention

The Nutrition Screening Initiative has adopted a basic consensus position on options for intervention in the prevention, reduction of risk factors, and management of poor nutritional status:

■ There exists a range of useful nutrition interventions all along the continuum of care.

■ These interventions exist both in the context of preventive and clinical care.

■ While there clearly is need for additional research in the efficacy of various interventions, nutrition is an important component of good health and medical practice.

While it is not an aim of the Initiative to reach consensus on specific interventions, we realize that screening will not prove useful unless interventions are available that can be readily implemented. *Screening Older Americans' Nutritional Health: Current Practices and Future Possibilities* by Johanna Dwyer, DSc, RD details a wide range of interventions. Included among these possibilities are:

■ Nutrition education, which can itself be an intervention, helping older Americans learn how to make healthier nutrition choices

■ Referral to and participation in various congregate and home-delivered meal programs funded under Title III of the Older Americans Act as well as other similar programs that may be available on a community basis

■ Referral for dental care when poor dentition or other oral health problems impede food consumption

■ Preparation of and counseling for diets to ensure adequate intakes of vitamins, minerals, protein, and energy and to control diabetes mellitus or other chronic diseases with dietary implications

■ Counseling or treatment for active alcoholics

■ Physical activity and exercise regimens

■ General referral to community support programs, whether in the public or private sector, that can provide:

- ❍ assistance with shopping or meal preparation
- ❍ social interaction and support to combat isolation
- ❍ assistance with transportation needs to facilitate food acquisition

■ Provision of special diets for institutionalized older adults that can be beneficial in the treatment of various chronic conditions

■ Special feeding routes involving parenteral and enteral nutrition for individuals who are unable to eat orally

By no means exhaustive, this list serves to highlight several key interventions that are widely understood and practiced. They reflect the fact that interventions may be provided by a variety of nonprofessional caregivers as well as by social services and health care professionals in various settings. Please take the time to investigate available resources in your community that could help older Americans improve their nutritional status.

Nutrition Screening Initiative

The Nutrition Screening Initiative is a five-year, multifaceted effort to promote routine nutrition screening and better nutrition care in America's health care system. Its initial focus is on older adults, one of the largest groups of Americans at risk of poor nutrition. The Initiative is a project of the American Academy of Family Physicians, The American Dietetic Association, and the National Council on Aging, Inc. A Blue Ribbon Advisory Committee of 27 key organizations and professionals from the fields of nutrition, medicine, and aging also plays an important role in guiding the effort.

In addition to developing the Checklist and screening tools found in this manual, the Initiative's Partners and Technical Review Committee have prepared a series of reports that review existing literature on nutrition and aging, identify the major risk factors associated with poor nutritional status, suggest major and minor indicators of poor nutritional status, and explain the Initiative's approach to nutrition screening. If you would like to learn more about nutritional issues in older adults or would like to receive these reference documents, full copies and executive summaries can be ordered from the Nutrition Screening Initiative.

Screening Older Americans' Nutritional Health: Current Practices and Future Possibilities
Johanna T. Dwyer, DSc, RD
Frances Stern Nutrition Center
Tufts University Medical School

Report of Nutrition Screening I: Toward a Common View
Consensus Conference
April 8-10, 1991

Includes the following papers:

Risk Factors Associated with Poor Nutritional Status in Older Americans
Jane V. White, PhD, RD
University of Tennessee at Knoxville

Indicators of Poor Nutritional Status in Older Americans
Richard J. Ham, MD
SUNY Health Science Center at Syracuse, NY

Development of an Approach to Nutrition Screening for Older Americans
David A. Lipschitz, MD, PhD
Little Rock VA Hospital
University of Arkansas for Medical Sciences

The Nutrition Screening Initiative welcomes your feedback in its effort to create a practical approach to nutrition screening and nutrition-related interventions. Comments on whether you have found the manual helpful, what you would like added or deleted from the current tools, and how you use them would be most appreciated. Please contact the Initiative at:

THE NUTRITION SCREENING INITIATIVE
2626 Pennsylvania Avenue, NW
Suite 301
Washington, DC 20037
(202) 625-1662

The Nutrition Screening Initiative is made possible in part through a grant from Ross Laboratories, a division of Abbott Laboratories.